Quality of Life

Quality of Life

Edited by

Alison J Carr

ARC Senior Lecturer in Epidemiology, University of Nottingham, Nottingham

Irene J Higginson

Professor of Palliative and Person Centred Care, Department of Palliative Care and Policy, Guy's, King's and St Thomas' School of Medicine, King's College London and St Christopher's Hospice, London

Peter G Robinson

Professor of Dental Public Health, Department of Oral Health and Development, School of Clinical Dentistry, University of Sheffield, Sheffield

BMJ
Books

SMC

© BMJ Books 2003
BMJ Books is an imprint of the BMJ Publishing Group

First published in 2003
by BMJ Books, BMA House, Tavistock Square,
London WC1H 9JR

www.bmjbooks.com

British Library Cataloguing in Publication Data

A catalogue record for this book is available from the British Library

ISBN 0 7279 1544 4

Typeset by SIVA Math Setters, Chennai, India
Printed and bound in Spain by GraphyCems, Navarra

Contents

Contributors

Julia Addington-Hall
Professor of Palliative Care, Research and Policy, Department of Palliative Care and Policy, Guy's, King's and St Thomas' School of Medicine, King's College London

Ann Bowling
Professor of Health Services Research, Department of Primary Care and Population Sciences, University College London

Alison J Carr
ARC Senior Lecturer in Epidemiology, University of Nottingham, Nottingham

Nora Donaldson
Honorary Senior Lecturer in Medical Statistics, Institute of Psychiatry, King's College London

Robert J Dunlop
Honorary Senior Lecturer, Department of Palliative Care and Policy, Guy's, King's and St Thomas' School of Medicine, King's College London

Bobbie Farsides
Senior Lecturer in Medical Ethics, Centre of Medical Law and Ethics, King's College London

Barry Gibson
Lecturer in Sociology and Informatics as Applied to Dentistry, Guy's, King's and St Thomas' School of Medicine, King's College London

Irene J Higginson
Professor of Palliative and Person Centred Care, Department of Palliative Care and Policy, Guy's, King's and St Thomas' School of Medicine, King's College London and St Christopher's Hospice, London

Lalit Kalra
Professor of Stroke Medicine, Department of Medicine, Guy's, King's and St Thomas' School of Medicine, King's College London

Peter G Robinson
Professor of Dental Public Health, Department of Oral Health and Development, School of Clinical Dentistry, University of Sheffield, Sheffield

Jane K Seale
Lecturer in Assistive Technology and Co-ordinator of Masters in Assistive Technology, Centre of Rehabilitation Engineering, King's College London

David Sulch
Consultant Physician in Elderly Care, Department of Adult Medicine, Queen Elizabeth Hospital, London

Alan R Turner-Smith
Reader in Rehabilitation Engineering, Department of Medical Engineering and Physics, King's College London

Kelly A Vincent
PhD student, Department of Academic Rheumatology, Guy's, King's and St Thomas' School of Medicine, King's College London

1: Current state of the art in quality of life measurement

ANN BOWLING

Summary points

- The aim of including quality of life in health outcome indicators is to be responsive to patients' evaluations of their treatment and outcome.
- Quality of life is a collection of interacting objective and subjective dimensions. Quality of life is a dynamic concept; its parts also affect each other as well as the sum.
- Psychological concepts used to denote quality of life have potential roles as influences, constituents or mediators of perceived life quality.
- Quality of life in relation to health has traditionally been based on a "pathology" model of health and dependency, and has focused on the measurement of physical and mental decline, impaired role and social functioning.
- Broader measurement scales of health status are frequently used to measure quality of life. Rarely is the use of such scales as mere proxy measures of quality of life acknowledged or justified by investigators.
- It has yet to be confirmed whether individualised measures provide more reliable and valid measures of quality of life than standardised measures.

Defining quality of life

The measurement of health-related quality of life as an endpoint in health services research provides a subjective dimension to health status assessment. The intention is to be responsive to patients' evaluations of their treatment and outcome. However, quality of life (QoL) is an amorphous concept. While the term "quality" implies the degree of excellence of a characteristic, different people may value different areas of life, and therefore quality of life means different things to different people.

A broad range of, often overlapping, models of quality of life has been developed. These range from the needs and satisfaction-based models used widely in the evaluation of mental health services, models of life satisfaction, social wellbeing and social network employed in social gerontology, and psychological models which emphasise personal growth, control over life, cognitive competence and adaptability.[1] In relation to the latter, Zizzi et al. (1998)[2] pointed to the confusion surrounding the many psychological concepts commonly used to denote quality of life, with their potential roles as influences, constituents or mediators of perceived life quality. They argued that perceived quality of life is likely to be *mediated* by several interrelated variables, including self-related constructs (for example, self-mastery and self-efficacy, morale and self-esteem, perceived control over life) and these perceptions are likely to be *influenced* by cognitive mechanisms (for example, expectations of life, social values, beliefs, aspirations, and social comparison standards). Although the model is attractive, there is still little empirical data to support or refute the distinction between psychological constructs as mediating or influencing variables.

Quality of life in relation to health, or "health-related quality of life", has traditionally been based on a "pathology" model of health and dependency, and has focused on the measurement of physical and mental decline, impaired role and social functioning. In short, it has tapped the individual's performance of activities that are essential for the continuing functioning of the wider society (the model of "functionalism"). This approach has led to a negative focus in measurement, at the expense of the positive (for example, scales have been developed to measure levels of functional 'dis'abilities, rather than balanced scales with equal measures of levels of ability).[1] Descriptive and evaluative research based on negative models inevitably underestimates the quality of life of people. A different approach to definition has conceptualised health-related quality of life as the gap between present health and functional status and one's aspirations for these ("gap" theory).[3,4] This model is based on social expectations and comparisons with others. While innovative attempts have been made to operationalise and measure this gap,[4] there is little supporting evidence of the content validity of this model.

Recognition of the need for broader, more positive and balanced definitions of quality of life has resulted in more general adoption of the WHO Quality of Life Group's (WHOQOL) definition: "... an individual's perception of their position in life in the context of the culture and value systems in which they live and in relation to their goals, expectations, and standards and concerns. It is a broad-ranging concept affected in a complex way by the person's physical health, psychological state, level of independence, social relationships, and their relationships to salient features of their environment."[5] It is also a concept that is dependent on the perceptions of individuals. Research has cast doubt on the power of objective variables alone in predicting quality of life ratings, especially in view of the paradox of wellbeing (the presence of subjective wellbeing in the face of objective difficulties that would be expected to predict unhappiness).[6]

In short, quality of life is a collection of interacting objective and subjective dimensions. Quality of life is also a dynamic concept; values and self-evaluations of life may change over time in response to life and health events and experiences. Each area of quality of life can also have knock on effects on the others. For example, retaining independence and social participation may promote feelings of emotional wellbeing, but are partly dependent on retaining health and adequate finances. These can also be influenced by local transport facilities, type of housing, community resources, and social relationships. Quality of life is multidimensional and its parts affect each other as well as the sum. It poses inevitable challenges for measurement.

Measuring quality of life in healthcare

If a measurement scale is to be of value in clinical and population health research, it needs to be conceptually clear, valid, sensitive, and responsive to clinically significant change over time, reliable, to have an identified factor structure, and its scoring system needs to be interpretable. It needs to be acceptable to respondents and population norms should be available for the instrument. Of equal importance is researcher and respondent burden: the length of time it takes to complete, whether it can be self-completed rather than interviewer administered, and the ease with which it can be analysed. The process of developing measurement scales, and the assessment of quality of life, is not only a methodological challenge for investigators, but can also be taxing for respondents. Making an overall judgement about the quality of one's life implies a cognitive, intellectual activity and requires the complex assessment of one's experiences and priorities.[7] These priorities can also change over time, perhaps influenced by experience in life, and by changing values in response to life and health events ("response shift"). Measurement scales need to be sensitive to this.

Consistent with the multidimensional nature of the concept, investigators have identified a wide range of measures to tap quality of life. These include measures of emotional wellbeing (for example, measured with indicators of life satisfaction and self-esteem), psychological wellbeing (for example, measured with indicators of anxiety and depression and a wide range of cognitive indicators), social wellbeing and roles (for example, measured with indicators of personal and wider social capital, including social support and activities), and physical health and functioning (for example, measured with scales of self-rated health status, disability or ability to perform activities of daily living).[1,8]

However, a pragmatic approach to quality of life often prevails in the health literature, and clarification of the concept is generally avoided. This avoidance is implicitly justified with reference to its abstract nature. Concepts, theories, and definitions of quality of life are unclear or inconsistent.[9] The selection of measurement scales then often appears ad hoc, and broader health status scales are frequently used to measure quality of life. Rarely is the use of such scales as mere proxy measures of quality of life acknowledged or justified by investigators. It is implicitly assumed that, as they measure physical, psychological, and social functioning they also measure quality of life (for example, the Sickness Impact

Profile,[10] the Nottingham Health Profile[11] and the Short-Form-36[12]). A wide range of "disease-specific" health-related quality of life scales has also been developed in order to enhance the sensitivity of outcome measures to particular conditions. But few are explicitly based on a concept or model of quality of life and, at best, they are composed of narrow mental, physical, and social functioning subscales alongside symptom checklists. The content validity of many standardised measures requires addressing. This needs testing far more rigorously with the populations to whom the scales are to be administered if meaningful measurement is to be achieved, and to enhance confidence that we are asking the right questions.

The complexity of conceptualising and measuring quality of life is due partly to its subjective nature.[13] It is also due to the failure among investigators to separate out its component parts into indicator and causal variables,[14] in addition to the mediating variables suggested earlier.[2] Quality of life is influenced by causal variables, and the level of quality of life manifests itself in indicator variables, but our traditional approach to its measurement has implicitly assumed only indicator variables.[14] As Fayers and Hand (2002)[14] implied, in their discussion of the distinction between these variables, an appreciation of these two types of variable may lead to more appropriate measurement scales. This is the next step that is needed in quality of life research.

In addition, while the division of quality of life into pre-defined individual components (for example, physical, psychological, and social functioning) is helpful for measurement purposes, this approach may not tap the most pertinent domains of people's perceptions of quality of life. Nor does it capture the subjectivity of people. Analyses of the public's perceptions of quality of life suggest that many domains prioritised by the public as important are not included in the most popularly used measures of quality of life, particularly in the health field.[15] Moreover, if measurement scales give equal weighting to the various subdomains of quality of life it is unlikely that the domains will have equal significance to different social groups or to individuals within these. Even where scales are weighted it is unlikely that the weightings will be equally applicable to different people.

The increasing focus on psychometric abilities in scale development, and the constant search for shorter measurement scales, carries the risk that areas of importance to large numbers of the populations of interest are omitted from questionnaires if they fail to "perform".

These problems have influenced the development of measures of the individual's perceptions of quality of life, and of their priorities. The approaches vary from the insertion of an "individualised" item into standardised lists of activities of daily living, which aims to tap the individual's values (for example, 'Which of these activities would you most like to be able to do without the pain or discomfort of your arthritis?');[16] open-ended items or scales identifying activities or important areas of life affected by the medical condition;[4,17–19] and open ended approaches asking people to identify and weight the important areas of their generic quality of life.[20] These individualised measures differ in their format, context (generic, health-related, disease-specific), complexity of administration, weighting, scoring, and psychometric properties. It is still unclear which of these is most reliable, valid, and suitable for measuring quality of life in the context of health, disease or generically. It is conceptually attractive to invite respondents to choose their own domains of quality of life and to weight these. But on a practical level, all individualised methods are relatively time consuming, require the help of an interviewer, and are more complex to analyse than standardised scales. There has been little research on whether these methods lead to any improvement in validity, sensitivity or specificity in comparison with the standardised scales. In addition, the data produced by individualised measures are presented at group level. Thus, Jenkinson and McGee (1998)[21] have questioned the assumption that this is acceptable, given that one might be "adding up apples and oranges (i.e. unrelated phenomena) rather than aspects of a single unitary concept of quality of life." Research is needed to compare the amount of explained variance in quality of life assessments achieved by individualised weighting and scoring methods, in comparison with standardised measures. The hypothesis that individualised measures provide more reliable and valid measures of quality of life than standardised measures has yet to be confirmed.[22]

In conclusion, these issues are all challenges for future methodological research. Quality of life research in healthcare has exploded into a relatively large industry over the past two decades. There are now hundreds of measures that are used to tap health-related or disease-specific quality of life. It is not a time to be complacent, but it is now timely to take stock and prepare to address the methodological challenges that have been identified.

References

1. Bowling A. *Measuring disease. A review of disease specific quality of life measurement scales, 2nd ed.* Buckingham: Open University Press, 2001.
2. Zizzi A, Barry MM, Cochrane R. A mediational model of quality of life for individuals with severe mental health problems. *Psychol Med* 1998;28:1221–30.
3. Calman KC. Quality of life in cancer patients: a hypothesis. *J Med Ethics* 1984;10:124–7.
4. Garratt AM, Ruta DA. The Patient Generated Index. In: Joyce CRB, O'Boyle CA, McGee H, eds. *Individual quality of life. Approaches to conceptualisation and assesment.* Amsterdam: Harwood Academic Publishers, 1999, pp. 105–18.
5. World Health Organization. *Measuring quality of life: the development of the World Health Organization Quality of Life Instrument* (WHOQOL). Geneva: WHO, 1993.
6. Mroczek DK, Kolarz CM. The effect of age on positive and negative affect: a developmental perspective on happiness. *J Pers Soc Psychol* 1998;75:1333–49.
7. Veenhoven R. Is happiness relative? *Soc Indicators Res* 1991; 24:1–34.
8. Bowling A. *Measuring health. A review of quality of life measurement scales, 2nd ed.* Buckingham: Open University Press, 1997.
9. Fitzpatrick R, Davey C, Buxton MJ, Jones, DR. Evaluating patient-based outcome measures for use in clinical trials. *Health Technol Assess* 1998;2(14).
10. Bergner M. Development, testing and use of the Sickness Impact Profile. In: Walker SR, Rosser RM, eds. *Quality of Life: Assessment and Application.* Lancaster: MTP Press, 1988.
11. Hunt SM, McEwan J, McKenna SP. *Measuring Health Status.* Beckenham: Croom Helm, 1986.
12. Ware JE, Snow KK, Kosinski M, Gandek B. SF-36 *Health Survey.* Boston, MA: New England Medical Centre, 1993.

13. Bowling A, Windsor J. Towards the good life. A population survey of dimensions of quality of life. *J Happiness Stud* 2001;**2**:55–81.
14. Fayers PM, Hand, DJ. Causal variables, indicator variables and measurement scales: an example from quality of life. *J R Stat Assoc* 2002;**165**(2):1–21.
15. Bowling A. What things are important in people's lives? A survey of the public's judgements to inform scales of health related quality of life. *Soc Sci Med* 1995;**10**:1447–62.
16. Tugwell P, Bombardier C, Buchanan WW *et al*. The MACTAR Patient Preference Disability Questionnaire. *J Rheumatol* 1987; **14**:446–51.
17. Guyatt GH, Berman LB, Townsend M *et al*. A measure of quality of life for clinical trials in chronic lung disease. *Thorax* 1987;**42**:773–8.
18. Guyatt GH, Nogradi S, Halcrow S *et al*. Development and testing of a new measure of health status for clinical trials in heart failure. *J Gen Intern Med* 1989;**4**:101–7.
19. Guyatt GH, Mitchell A, Irvine EJ *et al*. A new measure of health status for clinical trials in inflammatory bowel disease. *Gastronenterol* 1989;**96**:804–10.
20. Hickey A, O'Boyle CA, McGee HM, Joyce CRB. The Schedule for the Evaluation of Individual Quality of Life. In: Joyce CRB, O'Boyle CA, McGee H, eds. *Individual quality of life. Approaches to conceptualisation and assesment*. Amsterdam: Harwood Academic Publishers, 1999, pp. 119–34.
21. Jenkinson C, McGee H. *Health status measurement. A brief but critical introduction*. Oxford: Radcliffe Medical Press, 1998.
22. Fitzpatrick R. Assessment of quality of life as an outcome: finding measurements that reflect individuals' priorities (editorial). *Qual Health Care* 1999;**8**:1–2.

2: Is quality of life determined by expectations or experience?

ALISON J CARR, BARRY GIBSON AND
PETER G ROBINSON

Summary points

- Health-related quality of life is the gap between our expectations of health and our experience of it.
- We are disappointed if our experience does not match our expectations or we may be "pleasantly surprised" if our experience exceeds our expectations.
- Health-related quality of life therefore varies between and is dynamic within individuals.
- These concepts undermine current approaches in the measurement of health-related quality of life.
- People with different levels of expectation will report differing quality of life for the same clinical status.
- People with changing clinical status may report the same level of quality of life when the measures are repeated.
- Healthcare interventions may improve quality of life by restoring impairments or by adjusting expectations.
- Current quality of life measures do not take account of expectations and so cannot distinguish between changes in the experience of disease and changes in expectations of health.

Introduction

The way we think about health and healthcare is changing. Two factors driving this change are first, a recognition of the importance of the social consequences of disease and second, an acknowledgement that medical interventions aim to increase the quantity and quality of survival. For these reasons, the quality, effectiveness, and efficiency of healthcare are often evaluated by their impact on "quality of life".

There is no consensus definition of health-related quality of life but there is a tendency to regard it as a constant concept. Yet perceptions of health and its meaning vary between individuals and within an individual over time. This chapter argues that people assess their health-related quality of life by comparing their expectations with their experience of health. We propose a model for the relationship between expectations and experience and use it to illustrate current problems in quality of life measurement. The implications of these concepts for the use of quality of life as an indicator of treatment need and as an outcome of care will be discussed.

Definitions and determinants of health-related quality of life

Measures of health-related quality of life share a common theme; they summarise the judgements people make to describe their experiences of health and illness. This feature is what distinguishes them from measures of disability, which enquire about ability to complete specific tasks such as climbing stairs or dressing oneself. Health-related quality of life is a broader concept concerned with whether disease or impairment limits one's ability to fulfil a normal role (for example, whether the inability to climb stairs limits one at work). However, the measures do not consider how people arrive at these judgements. Understanding the mechanisms through which health, illness, and healthcare interventions influence quality of life (i.e. the determinants of health-related quality of life) may highlight ways in which quality of life can be maximised.

A major aim of treatment, particularly in chronic disease, is to enhance quality of life by reducing the impact of disease. Yet patients with severe disease do not necessarily report poor quality of life.[1] The relationship between symptoms and quality of life is therefore neither simple nor direct. Considering quality of life as the discrepancy between our expectations and experience provides a way of explaining how we evaluate our quality of life.[2]

Expectations, experience, and health-related quality of life

Our everyday lives are complex. When we are asked about them (whether in conversation or questionnaires) we need ways to simplify our thoughts to provide answers. We achieve this simplification by using expectations as sets of stabilised assumptions to inform our observations. A haematologist uses reference values to judge a blood sample in the same way. For example, someone with back pain may expect that consulting a doctor will solve their problem. They will have expectations about how they will be treated, the amount of pain to be encountered, and how effective their treatment will be.

A model of health-related quality of life

The model depicted in Figure 2.1 represents the relationship between expectations and experience of quality of life. Most quality of life measures detect the negative impact of disease or treatment on quality of life. When expectations are matched by current experience, there is no quantifiable impact on quality of life (period A). Whenever the experience of health falls short of expectations there is an impact (period C). The model demonstrates a number of possible trajectories in illness (Figure 2.1a-d). Impacts may resolve as the experience of health returns to the original level, illness may persist with continued disappointment in expectations, or we may be pleasantly surprised by the effectiveness of therapy.

Implications for the measurement of health-related quality of life

This model illustrates three problems in measuring health-related quality of life: that we will encounter people with

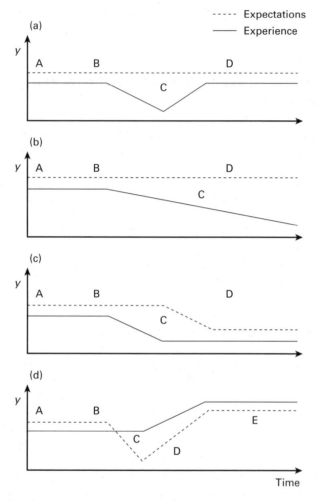

Figure 2.1 Four models of back pain occurring in a 35 year old woman at different times (A-E). In the figure (a) shows an acute episode; (b) shows a chronic episode; (c) shows her acceptance of a chronic condition; and (d) shows different effects of expectations and experience over time.

different levels of expectation; that we do not know the position of someone on their illness trajectory when we measure their quality of life; and that the reference value of expectation may change over time.

The first problem occurs because expectations are learned from experiences and are therefore highly specific. They vary between individuals, subject to differences in social, psychological, socio-economic, demographic, and other cultural factors. Expectations about quality of life are closely related to people's relationship with their environment. This may lead to structural variations in evaluations of impacts on quality of life. For example, older people have described the need to adapt to one's changing circumstances as a means of successfully coping with ageing.[3]

These variations in evaluation of impacts on quality of life can be incorporated into the model through the y axis and would be represented by something that helped to differentiate people with respect to their expectations and experiences. The result is that evaluations of quality of life are made within horizons of possibilities that people see for themselves and are therefore a fundamental component of their identity. These "horizons" of possibility are determined by factors such as social class, age, sex, ethnicity, sexuality, disability, and personal biography.

Existing measures of quality of life do not account for the levels of health expectations; they have no sense of the boundaries within which we measure levels of expectation and experience. The result is that someone with a poor health experience who has a low set of expectations for their health might not evaluate the experience as an impact on their quality of life because the boundaries of possibilities they expect are correspondingly low. Conversely someone who generally has good health might experience a significant impact on their quality of life from a relatively minor illness such as tonsillitis, because they have high health expectations. This problem may have very profound implications if quality of life measurements are to be used to prioritise and plan services, as has been proposed in dentistry.[4,5]

The second problem highlighted by the model is that the magnitude of the impact is dependent upon the point in time of the measurement. With existing quality of life measures it is impossible to ascertain at what point on the individual's disease trajectory the measurement has been made. Moreover, responses to illness are highly individualised; there is no standardised pattern followed by all patients. This means that even in a clinical trial where quality of life might be measured at equal intervals (and after the same duration of treatment) for all patients, they may still be at different points on different disease trajectories (such as those described in Figure 2.1).

The third problem arises because our experiences constantly change our expectations. In this respect we constantly move towards an ever-changing point of equilibrium. Psychological, sociological, and health services research all provide evidence that quality of life is a dynamic construct. The mechanisms with which people evaluate or quantify their quality of life change over time and in response to many factors.[6-11] The result is an inherent instability in the meaning it has for them.

This problem of "response shift" (i.e. that the terms of reference by which we judge change with time) is compounded if repeat measures are made over time, for example when we evaluate an intervention. For example, in Figure 2.1c if quality of life were measured at time point A and again at time point D using existing measures, no change in quality of life would be detected. This is because the period during which the impact occurred and expectations have changed has been missed. Therefore someone may have experienced an impact on their quality of life (at point C) and, although they have adapted to their changed health state through alterations in their expectations, they may still be considered to have a poorer life quality at point D than before their illness began at point A.

Implications for clinical practice

This model helps us understand how healthcare interventions may improve health-related quality of life and may allow us to increase the effect of treatment on quality of life. In the traditional model of healthcare, interventions restore impairments so that the experience of health returns to the original level of expectations.

Adaptation

The impact of chronic disease on quality of life can be minimised by helping patients to adjust their expectations and adapt to their changed clinical status. This approach is already adopted in many healthcare strategies including some psychological interventions, self-management programmes, and patient education groups.

One aim of assistive technology is to allow people to continue in their normal roles and meet their expectations of life despite their physical impairment and disability. Devices such as dentures and guide dogs help people bridge the gap between what they want to do and what their physical status allows them to do.

Expectations of treatment

As we have discussed previously, expectations are learned from experience. If previous episodes of back pain have settled after two days of sleeping on the floor, the expectation will be that a new episode will resolve in the same way. Likewise, experience of ineffective interventions may generate the expectation that new interventions will also be ineffective. These observations can be used to enhance the efficacy of treatment interventions. Significant success has been achieved in generating a response to both active and placebo interventions by changing negative expectations or creating positive expectations of treatment and health services.[12–16]

Conversely, unmet expectations are likely to result in dissatisfaction. Dissatisfied patients are more likely to experience a poor outcome through non-adherence to treatment regimens, by defaulting from follow up appointments, and by experiencing a poorer symptomatic response than satisfied patients.[17,18]

Implications for health promotion

Helping people to adapt to irreversible changes in their health status may be beneficial, but what should be done for those people whose expectations of health are unrealistically low?

Changing expectations of health is at the core of heath promotion. The experiences of some people cause them to have low expectations of health so that they accommodate significant levels of disease and disability. Health promotion is the process of helping people to take control over and improve their own health. The level of autonomy necessary for health promotion is possible only if people are aware of the possibilities open to them. Raising expectations of health is therefore an essential part of the "critical consciousness" of community development for health. In the drive to improve health, health promotion might increase the expectations of people with poor health and seemingly reduce their quality of life. This reflection on aspects of reality is part of the process of empowerment and provides the force that allows people to develop action to change that reality.[19]

Discussion and future issues

This model of health-related quality of life operationalises Calman's definition of quality of life as the gap between expectations and experience. It takes account of the fact that people see different possibilities for themselves when they evaluate impacts on their quality of life. Application of this model highlights some of the limitations of current methods of measuring quality of life in terms of their ability to assess accurately the impact of illness or treatment on quality of life, or their ability to quantify and understand changes in evaluations of impacts on quality of life over time. Further work is required to test the application of the model but the implications for the measurement of health-related quality of life are that significant modification of existing measures, the development of new measures, or analysis of the role of expectations and experience in quality of life-related evaluations are needed.

Acknowledgements

We thank our colleagues in the Interdisciplinary Research Group in Palliative and Person Centred Care at King's College

London, in particular Irene Higginson, Stanley Gelbier, Robert Dunlop, Julia Addington-Hall, Lalit Kalra, and Alan Turner-Smith, who have participated in discussions and commented on an earlier draft of this work. We also acknowledge the input and support of colleagues in the division of Dental Public Health and Oral Health Services Research at King's College London. Alison Carr's post is funded by the Arthritis Research Campaign.

References

1. Evans RW. Quality of life. *Lancet* 1991;**338**:363.
2. Calman KC. Quality of life in cancer patients: an hypothesis. *J Med Ethics* 1984;**10**:124–7.
3. MacEntee MI, Hole R and Stolar E. The significance of the mouth in old age. *Soc Sci Med* 1997;**45**:1449–58.
4. Ware JE, Brook RH, Davies AR, Lohr KN. Choosing measures of health status for individuals in general populations. *Am J Public Health* 1981;**71**:620–25.
5. Locker D. Applications of self–reported assessments of oral health outcomes. *J Dent Educ* 1996;**60**:494–500.
6. Allison PJ, Locker D, Feine JS. Quality of life: a dynamic construct. *Soc Sci Med* 1997;**45**:221–30.
7. Deiner E. Subjective well–being. *Psychol Bull* 1984;**95**:542–75.
8. Bunk B, Collins R, Taylor S, van Yperen N, Dakof G. The affective consequences of social comparison: either direction has its ups and downs. *J Pers Soc Psychol* 1990;**59**:1238–49.
9. Chamberlain K, Zika S. Stability and change in subjective well-being over short time periods. *Soc Indicators Res* 1992;**26**:101–17.
10. Englert JS, Ahrens B, Gebhardt R *et al*. Implications of the concepts of coping and quality of life for criteria of course and outcome. *Pharmacopsychiatrica* 1994;**27**:34–6.
11. Headey B, Holstrom E, Wearing A. The impact of life events and changes in domain satisfaction on well-being. *Soc Indicators Res* 1984;**15**:203–27.
12. Roberts AH, Kewman DG, Mercier L, Hovell M. The power of non-specific effects in healing: implications for psychological and biological treatments. *Clin Psychol Rev* 1993;**13**:375–91.
13. Thomas KB. General practice consultations: is there any point in being positive? *BMJ* 1987;**294**:1200–2.
14. Hashish I, Ho KH, Harvey W, Feinmann C, Harris M. Reduction of postoperative pain and swelling by ultrasound treatment: a placebo effect. *Pain* 1988;**33**:303–11.

15. Freund J, Krupp G, Goodenough D, Preston LW. The doctor–patient relationship and drug effect. *Clin Pharmacol Ther* 1971; **13**:172–80.
16. Rabkin JG, McGrath PJ, Quitkin FM *et al*. Effects of pill-giving on maintenance of placebo response in patients with chronic mild depression. *Am J Psychiatry* 1990;**147**:1622–6.
17. Ross CK, Frommelt G, Hazelwood L, Chang RW. The role of expectations in patient satisfaction with medical care. *J Health Care Marketing* 1987;**7**:16–26.
18. Becker MH, Maimon LA. Strategies for enhancing patient compliance. *J Community Health* 1980;**6**:113–35.
19. Freire, P. *Pedagogy of the oppressed*. Harmondsworth: Penguin, 1972.
20. Greer S. The psychological dimension in cancer treatment. *Soc Sci Med* 1984;**18**:345–9.
21. Bullinger M, Anderson R, Cella D, Aaronson N. Developing and evaluating cross-cultural instruments from minimum requirements to optimal models. *Qual Life Res* 1993;**2**:451–9.

3: Are quality of life measures patient-centred?

ALISON J CARR AND IRENE J HIGGINSON

Summary points

- Quality of Life is an individual construct and measures should take account of this.
- Many widely used measures of quality of life are not patient-centred because of their underlying constructs, the ways in which items were generated and chosen for inclusion in the questionnaire, the structure of the questionnaire restricting patient choice, and the system of weighting used.
- This limitation compromises their accuracy and utility because they are not measuring what constitutes quality of life to all patients.
- It is possible to measure QoL in a patient-centred way using individualised measures and these are receiving increasing interest.
- Some of the newer standardised quality of life measures may be more patient-centred than their predecessors but establishing this requires further research.

Introduction

Quality of life measures are increasingly used to supplement objective (clinical or biological) measures of disease in assessments of the quality of services, healthcare need, effectiveness, and cost-utility. This reflects a growing appreciation of the importance of how patients feel, how satisfied they are with treatment, and of disease outcomes.

In this respect, quality of life measures are seen as ways of capturing patients' perspectives of their disease and treatment, their perceived need for healthcare, and their preferences for treatment and disease outcomes. They are hailed as being "patient-centred". But the challenge in measuring quality of life lies in its uniqueness to individuals. Many of the existing measures of quality of life fail to take account of this, imposing standardised models of quality of life and pre-selected domains, which make them measures of general health status rather than quality of life. Are such measures truly patient-centred? To what extent do they really represent the quality of life of individual patients or groups of patients? Are they simply descriptions of patients' health status in relation to health professionals' or society's idea of what quality of life ought to constitute for people who are ill, which may include things that have little relevance or importance for patients?

This chapter explores another issue relating to the measurement of quality of life; the extent to which standardised quality of life measures accurately quantify quality of life in individual patients. It will debate whether newer approaches that are individualised and allow patients to define their quality of life in relation to their goals and expectations are more appropriate.

Arguments for the individual nature of quality of life

Although there is no single, agreed definition of health-related quality of life, quality of life is usually regarded as being relative to individual or cultural expectations and goals (Box 3.1). Chapter 2 proposes a model of quality of life that takes account of the interaction between expectations and experience. Whilst it seems reasonable to assume that there are some aspects of life that are of universal relevance to quality of life, the specific weights that individuals attach to these will differ between and within different cultural settings. Other aspects may be exclusively important to individuals. For example, Chapter 2 considers how the variations that exist between groups and individuals in expectations of health will impact on the measurement of quality of life. The interactions between all these aspects (generic and individual) will also vary between individuals.[1] Moreover, these factors and their interrelationships are unlikely to remain static over time.[2]

Values and priorities change in response to life circumstances (such as a life-threatening illness) and experience (such as ageing or adaptation to chronic illness). Viewed in this way, both the determinants and evaluations of quality of life are highly individual.

Box 3.1 Definitions of quality of life

Quality of life is determined by:

- the extent to which hopes and ambitions are matched by experience[3]
- individuals' perceptions of their position in life taken in the context of the culture and value systems where they live and in relation to their goals, expectations, standards, and concerns[4]
- appraisal of one's current state against some ideal[5]
- the things people regard as important in their lives.[6]

Evidence for the individual nature of quality of life

Attempts to quantify and compare quality of life across different populations of patients using standardised, generic measures have been confounded by the so-called "disability paradox". Patients who clearly have significant health and functional problems or intrusive symptoms do not necessarily produce quality of life scores commensurate with their health state. More than half of patients with moderate to severe disabilities report an excellent or good quality of life, despite experiencing severe difficulties performing daily tasks, being socially isolated and receiving limited incomes and benefits.[3] Transplant patients, haemodialysis patients, and peritoneal dialysis patients who report a wide variety of health problems are more likely to rate themselves as "very happy" than the general population,[4] and patients with neoplasms rate their quality of life in the top quartile of the WHOQOL questionnaire across all life domains (better than all other groups of patients including those attending a family planning clinic).[5]

These discrepancies are replicated at the level of the individual patient. Several studies have demonstrated the disparity between patients', doctors', and relatives' ratings of the patient's quality of life[6,7] or have suggested that doctors are unsuccessful in identifying aspects of disease and treatment of importance to patients.[8,9] The implications of these findings for the use of proxies to measure patients' quality of life will be discussed in Chapter 6, "Who should measure quality of life?"

These data provide evidence for the individual weighting of generic factors influencing quality of life and the presence of other factors important to quality of life that are not included in standardised quality of life measures. They also suggest that quality of life is a dynamic construct that alters in response to illness.

Are existing measures patient-centred?

Content

The lack of a widely agreed definition of health-related quality of life means that many of the existing measures are not based on any underlying theoretical conceptualisation of quality of life. Those few measures that are based on a theoretical model of quality of life such as the Patient Generated Index,[10] the Repertory Grid,[11] and the World Health Organization quality of life measures WHOQOL-100[5] and WHOQOL-BREF, are not widely used. This has led questionnaire developers to employ a variety of sources for the content of their questionnaires. Many earlier quality of life questionnaires were based on health professionals' definitions of what was relevant to quality of life. Some were based on reviews or adaptations of existing scales (such as EuroQol,[12] the McMaster Health Index,[13] and the SF-36[14]). Few directly asked patients about those factors that constituted quality of life. Where they did involve patients, they asked about the impact of illness on people's lives or behaviours (for example, the Nottingham Health Profile[15] and the Sickness Impact Profile[16]) but not about the important things in life. The result is that there is a danger that most of the widely used measures do not address what is important to patients in determining their quality of life. One illustration of this is that the most important factor influencing the reported quality of life of cancer patients attending an outpatient clinic was not being able to find a parking place each time they came to the clinic, something that was not addressed in any of the quality of life measures used.[17] Further evidence for the limitations of quality of life measures in capturing what is important or relevant to patients comes from qualitative and survey research of the quality of life of different patient groups.[18,19] When the quality of life domains identified in these studies are compared with the domains captured by some of the most widely used measures (Table 3.1), it is clear that, whilst there is some overlap (in the generic quality of life factors), there are factors of importance to patients that are not captured by quality of life measures, and factors included in quality of life measures that may be redundant or irrelevant to patients.

Weighting the importance of the domains

Quality of life has many distinct but related determinants, some of which are captured in separate domains in quality of life measures. Scoring involves either recording the quality of life for each domain separately (profile measures) or combining the results from all domains to give a composite quality of life score (index measures). Meaningful interpretation of the results would be easier if there were some estimate of the relative importance of each of these domains. For example, pain is included in the physical domain of most quality of life measures but the importance attached to it varies across cultures.[20]

Existing quality of life measures have approached this problem in different ways. Some measures do not include any weighting on the basis that patients find it impossible to value comparatively important life domains such as their family relationships and their ability to work. Others have used weights derived from the general or patient populations who are asked to value the range of health states included in the questionnaire. Patients' responses are then valued according to these weights. However, these are unlikely to represent individual patients' values. Different patient groups attach a range of weights to the same and different domains of importance (between patient variation)[21] and the weights

Table 3.1 Domains included in selected quality of life questionnaires or mentioned by patients as being important

Domain	Questionnaires			Patients' responses		
	SF-36[19]	EuroQol[17]	NHP[20]	OPCS omnibus patients[6]	Rheumatoid arthritis patients[23]	Neuromuscular disease patients*
Pain	Yes	Yes	Yes	Yes	Yes	Yes
Energy or tiredness	Yes	Not included	Yes	Yes	Not mentioned	Yes
Sleep	Not included	Not included	Yes	Not mentioned	Not mentioned	Not mentioned
Physical functioning or mobility	Yes	Yes	Yes	Yes	Yes	Yes
Daily living activities	Yes	Yes	Yes	Yes	Yes	Yes
Social interactions	Yes	Not included	Yes	Yes	Yes	Yes
Leisure activities	Yes	Yes	Not included	Not mentioned	Yes	Yes
Relationships	Not included	Not included	Not included	Yes	Yes	Yes
Sexual functioning	Not included	Not included	Not included	Yes	Yes	Not mentioned
Work	Yes	Not included	Not included	Yes	Yes	Yes
Emotional wellbeing	Yes	Yes	Yes	Yes	Yes	Yes
Dependence or independence	Not included	Not included	Yes	Not mentioned	Yes	Yes
Self perception or body image	Not included	Not included	Not included	Not mentioned	Yes	Yes
Perceptions of the future	Not included	Not included	Not included	Not mentioned	Yes	Yes

SF-36 = Medical outcomes study 36 item short form health survey; EuroQol = European quality of life measure; NHP = Nottingham health profile; OPCS = Office of Population, Censuses, and Surveys.
* Information from personal communication from K Vincent and M Rose, 1999.

patients attach to the same domains at different periods in their treatment and recovery change (within patient variation).[22] In the same way that the determinants of quality of life are specific to individuals, the importance attached to those determinants will be influenced by individual expectations and aspirations as well as their individual and cultural belief systems and socio-demographic factors such as age, gender, socio-economic status, education, geographical location, and marital status. A true assessment of quality of life can only be achieved using individual patient weights.

Does it matter if existing measures are not patient-centred?

Using quality of life measures that are not patient-centred can result in a number of problems:

- If they do not cover domains of quality of life of importance to individual patients they may not be valid measures of quality of life for those patients. Thus, standardised quality of life measures (where the questions and range of answers are pre-determined and the same for all patients) may measure something distinct from the quality of life of individual patients. In Bowling's study[19] there were discrepancies between patients' free response answers about areas of life most affected by disease and those elicited using prompt cards, further suggesting that results obtained using standardised measures may not capture patients' quality of life.
- If such measures are not capturing the quality of life of individual patients, they are unlikely to be responsive to change following treatment interventions (because they may not be measuring what is important to the patient) and their scores may be difficult to interpret.
- Quality of life measures that are not patient-centred differ in content and the weights or importance they apply to different domains. This can result in significantly different quality of life scores obtained from the same intervention in the same patients. The SF-36 and EuroQol, both standardised measures of quality of life, produced contradictory results in assessing the effectiveness of

cosmetic surgery in the same patients.[23] This clearly has implications for the use of non patient-centred quality of life measures in determining the effectiveness of interventions, the relative quality of services or to guide the allocation of resources.

Individualised measures

It is possible to measure quality of life in a patient-centred way using individualised measures (Box 3.2). Although less widely used than standardised measures, these are receiving increasing interest. However, they have their own problems. First, some patients have difficulty understanding the system of direct weighting, which limits their use as self-completed questionnaires[24] among patients who are very sick or among those who have compromised concentration spans for any reason. Second, patients may not readily volunteer some important aspects, particularly those related to mood,[25] and the information that an individual is willing to volunteer may change over time.[26] Finally, because of its individualised nature, interpretation and analysis of some of the data is complex. This can make comparison of groups of patients or change within individuals over time difficult, although many of the measures take account of this by using specific change questions. Further work is needed to refine and evaluate these individualised measures.

Discussion and future issues

Many of the widely used measures of quality of life are limited in their ability to capture the quality of life of individual patients. These limitations result from the structure and content of the measures, the ways in which they were developed and their systems of weighting. Some of these problems can be overcome by individualised measures but these have their own problems, which need further attention. A compromise may be the use of recently developed standardised measures, which are sufficiently broad to include

---

Box 3.2 Individualised measures of quality of life and health status

- The schedule for the evaluation of individualised quality of life (SEIQOL) is a questionnaire administered by an interviewer.[1] Patients are asked to specify the five areas of their life that are most important and then rate their current status in each of these areas using a visual analogue scale that ranges from 0 to 100. In the direct weighting version patients are then asked to rate the relative importance of each of the areas using a sectogram (a cardboard pie chart in which the size of the slices can be varied manually). Results can be presented as a profile of the five areas (in a bar chart) or as a global score.
- The Patient Generated Index (PGI)[9] is based on Calman's definition of quality of life as being the extent to which hopes and ambitions are matched by experience.[3] It can be administered by an interviewer or self-administered, although some problems have occurred with the postal, self-administered version. Patients specify the five areas of their life that are most affected by their condition. They then rate how badly affected they have been in these areas on a visual analogue scale that ranges from 0 to 100. Patients then weight the relative importance of these areas by allocating a total of 60 "spending points" between them: the most points are allocated to the area in which an improvement in health would be most important. The severity ratings are multiplied by the proportion of points allocated to an area and combined to give an index ranging between 0 and 100.
- The disease repercussion profile (DRP) assesses the impact of disease, the personal consequences of that impact, and the importance of these consequences in each of six areas of life: functional activities, social activities and interactions, relationships, finance or work, emotional wellbeing, and body image and self-esteem.[18] It produces a profile of the impact of the disease on quality of life. The profile is a self-completed measure originally designed specifically for clinical practice but it has also been used successfully in clinical trials and cross-sectional surveys.

most facets of life important to any patient and use direct weighting systems so that the result is an individualised assessment of quality of life (Box 3.3). The extent to which such measures reflect individual quality of life requires further assessment and their clinical utility and interpretability need to be established.

Box 3.3 Standardised measures for capturing an individual's quality of life

- The subjective quality of life profile (SQLP) is a self-administered, predefined checklist that covers a broad range of domains (functional, social, material, spiritual) and assesses an individual's goals including the importance attributed to the goal, tolerance of the distance between reality and the goal, and the ability to cope with this distance.[31] It produces a profile of quality of life.
- The World Health Organization's quality of life profile (WHOQOL-100) was developed by the WHO as a multilingual, multidimensional profile of quality of life for cross-cultural use.[9] The UK version is self-administered and covers 25 facets of quality of life within six broad domains. It assesses domains of satisfaction with life as well as the impact of disease or illness, and it captures positive and negative aspects of quality of life.

Acknowledgements

We thank our colleagues in the Interdisciplinary Research Group in Palliative and Person Centred Care at King's College London, in particular Peter Robinson, Barry Gibson, Stanley Gelbier, Robert Dunlop, Julia Addington-Hall, Lalit Kalra, and Alan Turner-Smith, who have participated in discussions and commented on an earlier draft of this work. Alison Carr's post is funded by the Arthritis Research Campaign.

References

1. Bernheim JL. How to get serious answers to the serious question: "How have you been?": subjective quality of life (QOL) as an individual experiential emergent construct. *Bioethics* 1999; **13**:272–87.
2. O'Boyle CA, McGee H, Hickey A, O'Malley K, Joyce CRB. Individual quality of life in patients undergoing hip replacement. *Lancet* 1992;**339**:1088–91.
3. Albrecht GL, Devlieger PJ. The disability paradox: high quality of life against all odds. *Soc Sci Med* 1999;**48**:977–88.
4. Evans RW. Quality of life. *Lancet* 1991;**338**:363.
5. Skevington S. Measuring quality of life in Britain: introducing the WHOQOL-100. *J Psychosom Res* 1999;**47**:449–59.

6. Slevin ML, Plant H, Lynch D, Drinkwater J, Gregory WM. Who should measure quality of life, the doctor or the patient? *Br J Cancer* 1988;**57**:109–12.

7. Pearlman RA, Uhlmann RF. Quality of life in chronic diseases: perceptions of elderly patients. *J Gerontol* 1988;**43**:25–30.

8. Donovan J. Patient education and the consultation: the importance of lay beliefs. *Ann Rheum Dis* 1991;**50**:418–21.

9. Kwoh K, Feinstein A, Gifford R *et al*. Physician-patient agreement on patients' priorities for important treatment outcomes. *Arthritis Rheum* 1987;**30**(suppl 4):101.

10. Ruta DA, Garratt AM, Leng M, Russell IT, MacDonald LM. A new approach to the measurement of quality of life: the Patient-Generated Index. *Med Care* 1994;**32**:1109–26.

11. Thunedborg K, Allerup P, Bech P, Joyce CRB. Development of the Repertory Grid for measurement of individual quality of life in clinical trials. *Int J Methods in Psychiatr Res* 1993;**3**:45–56.

12. Euroqol Group. *Euroqol EQ-5D User Guide*. Rotterdam Centre for Health Policy and Law, Erasmus University, 1996.

13. Chambers LW. *The McMaster Health Index Questionnaire (MHIQ): methodologic documentation and report of second generation of investigators*. Hamilton, ON: McMaster University, Dept Clinical Epidemiology and Biostatistics, 1982.

14. Ware JE, Sherbourne CD. The MOS 36-item Short-form Health Survey (SF-36) I. Conceptual framework and item selection. *Med Care* 1992;**30**:473–83.

15. Hunt SM, McEwan J, McKenna SP. *Measuring Health Status*. Beckenham: Croom Helm, 1986.

16. Bergner M, Bobbitt RA, Carter WB *et al*. The Sickness Impact Profile: development and final revision of a health status measure. *Med Care* 1981;**19**:787–805.

17. Coates AS, Kaye SB, Sowerbutts T *et al*. On the receiving end: patient perceptions of side-effects of cancer chemotherapy. *Eur J Clin Oncol* 1983;**13**:203–8.

18. Carr AJ. A patient-centred approach to evaluation and treatment in rheumatoid arthritis: the development of a clinical tool to measure patient-perceived handicap. *Br J Rheumatol* 1996;**35**: 921–32.

19. Bowling A. What things are important in people's lives? a survey of the public's judgements to inform scales of health related quality of life. *Soc Sci Med* 1995;**41**:1447–62.

20. Skevington SM. Investigating the relationship between pain and discomfort and quality of life, using the WHOQOL. *Pain* 1998; **76**:395–406.

21. Rose M, Scholler G, Klapp BP, Bernheim JL. Weighting dimensions in generic QOL questionnaires by Amamnestic

Comparative Self-Assessment: different weights in different diseases. *Qual of Life Res* 1998;**7**:655.

22. Hickey AM, Bury G, O'Boyle CA, O'Kelly F, Shannon W. A new short form individual quality of life measure (SEIQOL-DW): application in a cohort of individuals with HIV/AIDS. *BMJ* 1996;**313**:29–33.

23. Klassen A, Fitzpatrick R, Jenkinson C, Goodacre T. Contrasting evidence for the effectiveness of cosmetic surgery from two health-related quality of life measures. *J Epidemiol Community Health* 1999;**53**:440–41.

24. Macduff C, Russell E. The problem of measuring change in individual health-related quality of life by postal questionnaire: use of the patient-generated index in a disabled population. *Qual Life Res* 1998;**7**:761–9.

25. Vachon ML, Kristjanson L, Higginson I. Psychosocial issues in palliative care: the patient, the family, and the process and outcome of care. *J Pain Symptom Manage* 1995;**10**(2):142–50.

26. Higginson I, Priest P, McCarthy M. Are bereaved families a valid proxy of a patient's assessment of dying? *Soc Sci Med* 1994;**38**(4):553–7.

4: Quality of life in caregivers

DAVID SULCH AND LALIT KALRA

Summary points

- The majority of people with chronic disability live at home and are supported by informal caregivers, often spouses or other close family members.
- Despite the importance of measuring quality of life in carers for both health outcome research and developing clinical practice, very few tools are specific to this group.
- Commonly used tools fail to capture domains relevant to caregivers and those developed for use in caregivers lack adequate validation.
- It is becoming increasingly clear that healthcare decisions should be based on evaluation of patient outcome in the context of the effects that chronic disease or disability have on those around them.
- A lot is known about the determinants of quality of life for caregivers; the challenge is to develop quality of life measures that are specific, sensitive, and relevant to this group.

Introduction

The demographic changes towards an older population by 2020 will result in an increased prevalence of chronic diseases due to cardiac, pulmonary, and cerebrovascular causes as well as dementias, arthropathies, locomotor disorders, and cancers.[1] The majority of people with chronic disability live at home and often require assistance for basic activities such as feeding, dressing, and toileting. The bulk of this support is provided by informal caregivers, often spouses or other close family members.[2] This support is not without cost to individuals, and the physical, psychological, emotional, and social consequences of the caregiver role are becoming increasingly recognised.[3-5]

As promoting wellbeing is central to management of chronic disease in which cure, by definition, is not possible, quality of life measures are being used increasingly to complement disease-specific measures when assessing effectiveness of health interventions.[6,7] There is increasing awareness that measurement of quality of life in chronic disease should not be limited to patients but should extend to their caregivers who may also be suffering from the consequences of disease. Quality of life measurement in caregivers presents particular challenges, which are discussed in this chapter.

The burden of care

Much research and service input in rehabilitation has concentrated successfully upon patient-focused interventions to prevent mortality and reduce institutionalisation.[8] This has contributed to an increase in the number of disabled patients being managed at home. These patients often have major impairments of functional abilities. In a recent study, 59% of 518 chronic stroke patients within private households needed help with self-care activities and 88% needed help with household activities.[9] The burden of care for these patients is often borne by informal carers.

Although carer stress and quality of life are key issues in the long-term management of disabled patients, these are often not given the attention they deserve in health outcome research. Factors influencing caregiver quality of life may be different from those influencing quality of life in patients. For example, performance as a caregiver, satisfaction with care received by the patients, and adjustments to the caregiver's personal life are specific to carers' perceptions of self-worth. These problems are recognised in stroke and dementia literature, and many new studies incorporate an assessment of carer quality of life as an outcome measure.[10] Carers, especially elderly people, may have their own health problems and may suffer further physical ill-health because of lifting (backache, injury) or accidents.[11]

The unrelenting burden of caring results in depression in a high proportion of carers, which is frequently unrecognised.[12] In addition, carers may be required to make significant changes in their lifestyle such as giving up work (resulting in loss of income and self-esteem) or social pursuits.[13] Carers may show marked strain and greater than expected problems with sleep, emotional reactions, and social isolation.[14]

Most relatives who provide support have little respite: only a minority leave the patient unattended for all or part of the day. It is not uncommon for these carers to feel chronically exhausted and to develop feelings of guilt because of perceived failings in providing care. The situation at home for carers is further compounded by feelings of isolation, poor physical and emotional support, and "carer fatigue", which results in a diminished ability to provide care. Increasing stress levels and decreasing coping behaviour in patients and their carers have also been demonstrated to result in increased use of statutory resources in dependent patients.[15]

Despite the valuable contribution made by caregivers to supporting disabled patients, their needs and quality of life are often given low priority. A large survey of stroke practice in Britain has shown that less than 50% of carers are given enough information during the hospital phase of management despite being more keen than patients to know about management options and support groups.[16] Carers are more dissatisfied than patients about the quality of information given and the level of social and health services support after discharge.[17] In addition, interventions undertaken to improve caregiver understanding and quality of life are haphazard and poorly timed.[18] Studies suggest that given time to accept the caregiver role, carers are receptive to learning about chronic disability and cope better with the care of the disabled patient.[19]

Quality of life measures

Measurement of quality of life in carers has largely utilised the same generic instruments that are used in patients, principally because they are familiar, simple to use, and allow comparisons between groups. The SF-36 and EuroQol are the two most well known instruments, scoring the interviewee on a range of domains from physical functioning to social participation.[20,21] As these instruments were developed for use in patients they emphasise domains such as physical functioning and pain, which may have little relevance in carers. On the other hand, domains such as social functioning, vitality, and mental health (also included in standard tools) are applicable to carers but may need to be given greater weight than in patients. In-depth interviews with carers have demonstrated that finances, family relationships, disease progression in the patient, and spirituality are important contributors to their quality of life,[22] but are not measured by most standard quality of life tools. The differences in the determinants of quality of life between patients and carers limit the ability of standard instruments to measure quality of life in caregivers and there is a need to develop specific and sensitive tools that facilitate accurate assessment of quality of life in this group.

A number of studies have described attempts to develop quality of life scales that are relevant to caregivers.[23,24] These scales can be general or disease-specific. General measures (for example, the Health Utilities Index) are designed to be used across populations or different diseases, whilst disease-specific measures (for example, those for malignancy or amyotrophic lateral sclerosis) incorporate questions about aspects typically affected by a specific disease or condition.[25-27] Another approach is based on the acceptance that there is great variability in factors that influence quality of life in individual carers and there is no single generic tool that can be applied universally. This has led to the development of individualised measures of quality of life that ask subjects what is most important to them, and how well they think that aspect of their life is going. Tools such as the Schedule for the Evaluation of Individual Quality of Life (SEIQoL) have been used successfully in patients receiving palliative care and those with HIV-related disease.[28,29] These tools have also been used to assess quality of life in carers of patients with ALS and with Alzheimer's disease[22,30] and are likely to have increasing application to assess the quality of life of caregivers in other situations. None of the specific tools developed for assessing carer quality of life has undergone rigorous evaluation to date or is used in routine clinical practice.

Caregiver burden and quality of life

The concept of caregiver burden has been understood for many years and many scales exist that have been specifically designed for assessment of this area. One commonly used scale, the Caregiver Burden Inventory,[31] measures the burden across five different domains. These are physical, social, emotional and developmental burden, and time dependence. Other scales, such as the Relatives Stress Scale,[32] provide similar information. Caregiver burden essentially measures the actual amount of care provided by the caregiver to the patient. A large burden of care does not necessarily imply a reduced quality of life, although studies suggest a strong link between objective burden and quality of life.[3] The extent of the caring role may act to improve self-esteem in some carers, particularly those who have undergone role adjustments due to retirement, for example. Improved self-esteem is recognised to improve quality of life.[33] Thus, although high carer burden threatens quality of life in general terms, it still needs to be considered separately for an accurate assessment of the impact of disease on carer status.

Why measure quality of life in caregivers?

There are many important reasons for measuring the quality of life of caregivers. At a political level, measuring quality of life could be a means of obtaining resources for caregivers and raising awareness of the problem amongst the general public and policy makers. At a theoretical level, measuring caregivers' quality of life could provide information about models of health and those factors influencing health. At a practical level, measures of caregivers' quality of life could be used to evaluate the effectiveness of healthcare, to quantify the health of populations and identify healthcare needs, and to identify specific problems in individual patients in clinical practice.

At present, carer quality of life measurements remain largely a research tool and are increasingly used as an outcome measure in intervention studies to alleviate the burden of chronic disabling diseases such as stroke and dementia.[34,35] Caregiver quality of life measurements, taken before and after an intervention, are particularly important for interventions that may not change the severity of illness or level of disability in patients, but provide supportive care. These include interventions such as respite care, family group support and education, counselling and advisory services, many of which lack evidence of effectiveness, probably because of the choice of outcome indicators in studies to evaluate their effectiveness.[36,37]

It is likely that measurement of carer quality of life will also gain importance in routine clinical practice. In theory, it may be possible to prevent breakdown of the care arrangements in disabled patients living at home by monitoring quality of life in caregivers and using this as a proxy measure for the need to intervene with additional support before a crisis arises. However, research is needed to evaluate the feasibility and effectiveness of sequential measurements of quality of life in routine clinical practice and to determine threshold quality of life levels at which breakdown of a specific situation is imminent.

Discussion and future issues

Quality of life is a key concept in modern healthcare and should be used in conjunction with probabilities of clinical outcomes in research and clinical practice. Recent decades have seen the development and validation of several tools providing quick and reliable assessment of quality of life. Despite the progress to date, research into the best ways of measuring quality of life and its applications to clinical practice must still be prioritised. Meanwhile, attention must be focused on the quality of life of those caring for patients with chronic disability. It is a mistake to assess the patient alone without regard to the effects of their illness on those around them. Increasing use of quality of life measures in such individuals will better inform healthcare practice, and play an important role in decision making in the future.

References

1. Manton KG, Corder L, Stallard E. Chronic disability trends in elderly United States populations: 1982–94. *Proc Natl Acad Sci* 1997;**94**:2593–8.
2. Schofield H, Bloch S. Disability and chronic illness: the role of the family carer. *Med J Aust* 1998;**169**:405–6.
3. Hughes SL. Giobbie-Hurder A. Weaver FM. Kubal JD. Henderson W. Relationship between caregiver burden and health-related quality of life. *Gerontologist* 1999;**39**:534–45.
4. Schneider J, Murray J, Banerjee S, Mann A. EUROCARE: a cross-national study of co-resident spouse carers for people with Alzheimer's disease: factors associated with carer burden. *Int J Geriatr Psychiatry* 1999;**14**:651–61.
5. Low JT, Payne S, Roderick P. The impact of stroke on informal carers: a literature review. *Soc Sci Med* 1999;**49**:711–25.
6. Guyatt GH, Feeney DH, Patrick DL. Measuring health-related quality of life. *Ann Intern Med* 1993;**118**:622–9.
7. Felce D, Perry J. Quality of life: its definition and measurement. *Res Dev Disabilities* 1995;**16**:51–74.
8. Stroke Unit Trialists Collaboration. How do stroke units improve patient outcomes? A collaborative systematic review of the randomized trials. *Stroke* 1997;**28**:2139–44.
9. Kavanagh S, Knapp M, Patel A. Costs and disability among stroke patients. *J Public Health Med* 1999;**21**:385–94.
10. Williams LS. Health-related quality of life outcomes in stroke. *Neuroepidemiol* 1998;**17**:116–20.
11. Carod-Artal FJ, Egido-Navarro JA, Gonzalez-Gutierrez JL, Varela de Seijas E. Perceptions of long term overload in care givers of patients who have survived a stroke. *Rev Neurol* 1999;**28**: 1130–8.
12. Draper BM, Poulos CJ, Cole AM, Poulos RG, Ehrlich F. A comparison of caregivers for elderly stroke and dementia victims. *JAGS* 1992;**40**:896–901.
13. Jones DA, Peters TJ. Caring for elderly dependents: effects on the carers' quality of life. *Age Ageing* 1992;**21**:421–8.
14. Thommassen B, Aarsland D, Braekhus A *et al*. The psychosocial burden on spouses of the elderly with stroke, dementia and Parkinson's disease. *Int J Geriatr Psychiatry* 2002;**17**:78–84.
15. Baldock J, Ungerson C. A consumer view of new community care: the home care experience of a sample of stroke survivors and their carers. *Care in Place* 1994;**2**:27–32.
16. Wellwood I, Dennis MS, Warlow CP. Perceptions and knowledge of stroke among surviving patients with stroke and their carers. *Age Ageing* 1994;**23**:293–8.

17. Wellwood I, Dennis MS, Warlow CP. Patients' and carers' satisfaction with acute stroke management. *Age Ageing* 1995;**24**:519–24.

18. McGowan A, Braithwaite V. Stereotypes of emotional caregivers and their capacity to absorb information: the views of nurses, stroke carers, and the general public. *J Adv Nurs* 1992;**17**:822–8.

19. Braithwaite V, McGowan A. Care-givers emotional well-being and their capacity to learn about stroke. *J Adv Nurs* 1993; **18**:195–202.

20. McHorney CA, Ware JE Jr, Raczek AE. The MOS 36-Item Short-Form Health Survey (SF-36): II. Psychometric and clinical tests of validity in measuring physical and mental health constructs. *Med Care* 1993;**31**:247–63.

21. EuroQoL – a new facility for the measurement of health related QOL. The EuroQoL Group. *Health Policy* 1990;**16**:199–208.

22. Bromberg MB, Forshew DA. Comparison of instruments addressing quality of life in patients with ALS and their caregivers. *Neurol* 2002;**58**:320–22.

23. Gallego CF, Roger MR, Bonet IB *et al*. Validation of a questionnaire to evaluate the quality of life of non-professional caregivers of dependent persons. *J Adv Nurs* 2001;**33**:548–54.

24. Weitzner MA, Meyers CA, Steinbrucker S, Saleeba AK, Sandifer SD. Developing a care giver quality of life instrument: preliminary steps. *Cancer Pract* 1997;**5**:25–31.

25. Bell CM, Araki SS, Neumann PJ. The association between caregiver burden and caregiver health-related quality of life in Alzheimer disease. *Alzheimer Dis Assoc Disord* 2001:**15**;129–36.

26. Weitzner MA, Jacobsen PB, Wagner H, Friedland J, Cox C. The Caregiver Quality of Life Index – Cancer (CQOLC) scale: development and validation of an instrument to measure quality of life of the family caregiver of patients with cancer. *Qual Life Res* 1999;**8**:55–63.

27. Gelinas DF, O'Connor P, Miller RG. Quality of life for ventilator dependent ALS patients and their caregivers. *J Neurol Sci* 1998;**160**(suppl 1):134–6.

28. Campbell S, Whyte F. The quality of life of cancer patients participating in phase I clinical trials using SEIQoL-DW. *J Adv Nurs* 1999;**30**:335–43.

29. Hickey AM, Bury G, O'Boyle CA *et al*. A new short form individual quality of life measure (SEIQoL-DW): application in a cohort of individuals with HIV/AIDS. *BMJ* 1996;**313**:29–33.

30. Scholzel-Dorenbos CJ. Measurement of quality of life in patients with dementia of Alzheimer type and their caregivers: Schedule for the Evaluation of Individual Quality of Life. *Tijdschr Gerontol Geriatr* 2000;**31**:23–6. (Original published in Dutch with abstracts in English.)

31. Novak M, Guest C. Application of a multidimensional caregiver burden inventory. *Gerontologist* 1989;**29**:798–803.
32. Philp I, Goddard A, Connell NA *et al*. Development and evaluation of an information system for quality assurance. *Age Ageing* 1994;**24**:150–53.
33. Kermode S, MacLean D. A study of the relationship between quality of life, health and self-esteem. *Aust J Adv Nurs* 2001; **19**:33–40.
34. Mant J, Carter J, Wade DT, Winner S. Family support for stroke: a randomised controlled trial. *Lancet* 2000;**356**:808–13.
35. Fillet HM, Gutterman EM, Brooks RL. Impact of donepezil on caregiving burden for patients with Alzheimer's disease. *Int Psychogeriatr* 2000;**12**:389–401.
36. Forster A, Young J. Specialist nurse support for patients with stroke in the community: a randomised controlled trial. *BMJ* 1996;**312**:1642–6.
37. Dowswell G, Lawler J, Young J, Forster A, Hearn J. A qualitative study of specialist nurse support for stroke patients and caregivers at home. *Clin Rehabil* 1997;**11**:293–301.

5: Assessing quality of life in children

KELLY A VINCENT AND IRENE J HIGGINSON

Summary points

- The conceptual and practical difficulties involved in assessing quality of life in children have resulted in inadequate research into this important area.
- Quality of life questionnaires adapted from adult measures or that use an adult model of quality of life are inappropriate for use with children.
- The rapid physical and cognitive changes in childhood make it difficult to interpret apparent changes in quality of life.
- The assessments of parents or carers can complement child assessments of quality of life but should only be used as proxies for children who are very young or otherwise unable to complete measures themselves.
- Age-appropriate scales and interviews involving computers, pictures, and videos provide promising ways of assessing quality of life in children.

Introduction

Illness and its consequences affect the lives of children. However, children's experience of ill health, medical intervention, and the effects of these upon development and adjustment are not well understood. It is assumed that hospitalisation, intrusive medical procedures, the uncertainty of survival, and prospects of disability have a negative effect upon children. In order to understand these effects and improve paediatric healthcare it is important that we are able to assess children's quality of life effectively. A lack of conceptual models of health and quality of life in children has made it difficult to develop practicable, valid measures of child quality of life. This chapter explores the problems involved in assessing the quality of life of children with particular reference to these conceptual and practical problems and the approaches that have been taken to address them.

How does quality of life in children differ from quality of life in adults?

Unsurprisingly, the challenges in assessments of quality of life in children relate to their age. The implications of age can be considered in four categories:

- physical development
- developing concepts of quality of life
- cognitive development
- the content of instruments.

These categories are arbitrary and artificial rather than discrete entities. If we adopt the WHO definition of health as complete physical, psychological, and social wellbeing then the concept of health pertinent to a young person is in part defined by the ability to participate in appropriate physical and social activities.[1,2] These physical and social activities will change as the child develops and therefore the content of quality of life instruments should focus on these activities in a way that the child can understand. However, these categories will be used for the purposes of discussion.

Physical development

Physical development is one of the most predictable changes in young people. None the less, the rapid physical changes that take place during childhood present a particular challenge to quality of life researchers. They make it difficult to determine whether changes in quality of life are caused by improvement or deterioration in physical condition or whether such changes are masked by development or adaptation. The child has been described as "a moving target for whom levels of function in various dimensions and even the dimensions themselves change with age and developmental stage."[3] This problem undoubtedly complicates the task of capturing what has already been acknowledged as a dynamic construct.[4]

Developing concepts of quality of life

Many quality of life measures used with children are based on adult models of quality of life.[5] Measures adapted in this way are inappropriate not only because their content may not be relevant, but because of the differences between child and adult perceptions of and interactions with the world. Very different conceptions of quality of life are held in research relating to children, varying from the holistic and psychosocial, to the biomedical and disease-based (Box 5.1).[6,7] This lack of agreement about conceptual models of quality of life in children has made it difficult to develop practicable, valid measures of child quality of life. Qualitative research is required to elucidate the concepts of quality of life held by young people.

Box 5.1 Two alternative conceptualisations of quality of life in children

- Quality of life in young children has been found to be more about having "shiny hair or lots of friends" than about the functional tasks emphasised in many adult quality of life assessments.[1]
- Paediatric quality of life refers to those areas of a child's or adolescent's functioning that are directly affected by an illness or its treatment.[6]

Young people are not a homogeneous group and the meaning of quality of life and its relevant dimensions will change with age.[3] The implications of developmental change are well illustrated in the changing significance of independence over the course of childhood.

Children rely on adults for financial, emotional, and, in very young children, physical support. However, gaining independence from parents is an important part of growing up. The disruption of this process by the effects of illness and treatment is likely to have a negative influence upon quality of life that will only be detected if the content of quality of life instruments is directed at the relevant context.

The context of the child's life influences the meaning of questions about physical, social, and psychological functioning. For example, play is likely to be a good indicator of the physical and psychological effects of illness in very young children, whereas educational achievement may be more relevant in older children.[8] The importance of body image is also likely to change over the course of childhood. Many illnesses, such as cystic fibrosis, interrupt physical development and normal growth,[9] which means that body image is likely to be a particular concern in childhood illness. Similarly, the effects of cancer treatment, such as hair loss and weight gain may cause distress, particularly during adolescence when sexuality and social acceptance become increasingly important.[10]

Unfortunately, issues relevant to the developing child, such as body image and independence, are not incorporated into the scales of Table 5.1. This may be due to limited information about these issues, particularly compared to the widely accessible information about the more physical and functional effects of illness.

One method of overcoming problems brought about by changing concepts of quality of life is the use of more general assessments. The Quality of My Life scale (QOML) developed for Juvenile Rheumatoid Arthritis does not incorporate specific domains of life, but asks participants to make global ratings of their quality of life.[11] This generic approach can be a useful adjunct to functionally based measures, such as those that measure health status in the rheumatic diseases of childhood.[12]

Cognitive development

The reading level of the child and his or her ability to understand concepts and the way they are presented in instruments are critical, and yet many instruments rely on advanced reading levels.[6] Typical quality of life questionnaires for adults have a literacy level of 13–14 years, which makes them difficult for most children as well as many adults.[5] Even if the questions are understood, the scaling of questionnaires with the use of numbers or adjectival descriptors may present further problems. Not only must children understand the question but they are also required to match their response to a specific scale.

Beyond the matter of literacy there is the issue of concept comprehension. Young children may not understand the abstract concepts involved in quality of life research.[13] For example, the utility model of quality of life involves formulating abstract preferences between quantity and quality of life. These concepts are difficult for children to understand and the choices are commensurately difficult for them to make.[6] Similarly, concepts involving different time frames are difficult for younger children to grasp. For example, children have difficulty in understanding the concept "during the last week" and it may be better to ask children to recall how they have been since a particular event rather than during a chronological period.[14]

Simplified questionnaires and interviewer-administered assessments may overcome limitations in children's levels of literacy and comprehension. Pictorial representations of faces displaying different degrees of happiness or sadness are often incorporated into questionnaires for children.[11,15–17]

Other methods, such as the use of interactive video or computers, may also be useful.[5] Proposed methods of assessing children's quality of life include the use of a "three wishes" section in quality of life interviews.[15] Framing interview questions in this way may provide information about the child's aspirations, which is an important concept in quality of life research in adults.[18] Story-telling techniques may also provide an enjoyable and productive way of eliciting quality of life information.

One other point is that longitudinal research will be undermined if there are developments in an individual child's comprehension of questions that will affect the way he or she responds to the questions.

Instrument content

Much of the content of adult quality of life questionnaires is not relevant or appropriate for children. Some quality of life measures used in children have been crudely adapted through the omission of adult items, such as "household management" and the substitution of words, such as "school" for "work".[6,8] Questions about sexual functioning and relationships are inappropriate until mid- to late adolescence. Even at this point the nature of questions about these topics should differ considerably between adults and adolescents. Questions about work and parenting are equally inappropriate.

The emphasis should reflect the main areas of life in childhood.[19] As family and social relationships are very important to the wellbeing of children, scales should include items about family roles and activities and also relationships with parents and siblings.[20] Similarly, questions about life at school should cover relationships with peers and friends as well as the ability to keep up with schoolwork.[19]

Table 5.1 indicates that most existing scales focus on physical and symptom-related aspects of quality of life.[14,22] They do not incorporate school-related items. Only two of the scales have domains specifically devoted to social aspects of life and just one considers the influence of illness upon the family.[21,23,24]

Different scales for different stages of development

With the rapid changes that occur in childhood it is better to develop conceptual models of quality of life for different age groups. Scales arising from this work can take account of life context, stages of cognitive development, and increasing levels of independence, providing a good basis on which to develop new questionnaires.

Advances in the development of different kinds of scales for different age groups have involved the development of scales specifically for adolescents and scales such as the Child Asthma Questionnaires (CHAQs) (Table 5.1).[17,41] The CHAQs

Table 5.1 Quality of life measures for children

Questionnaire	Domains covered	Completed by
Generic scales The Child Health Questionnaire[45]	Activity Achievement Comfort Disorders Resilience/risks Satisfaction	Parent form: 5–18 years old Child form: 10–18 years old
Childhood Health and Illness Profile[25]	Activity Comfort Satisfaction Disorders Achievement Resilience	Adolescents 11–17 years old
Quality of Wellbeing Scale[22]	Physical symptoms Mobility Physical activity Functional status	Parents Adolescents
Disease-specific scales Quality of My Life Questionnaire (QOML)[11] (Rheumatic conditions)	Global quality of life Health-related quality of life Change of quality in life	Children 4–12 years old (or parents)
The Paediatric Rhinoconjunctivitis Quality of Life Questionnaire[14]	Nose symptoms Eye symptoms Practical problems Other problems Activities	Children 6–12 years old
Paediatric Oncology Quality of Life Scale[33]	Physical function and role restriction Emotional distress Treatment-related adjustment	Parents of children 4–18 years old
The Paediatric Cancer Quality of Life Inventory–32 (PCQL–32)[23]	Disease and treatment related symptoms/problems Physical functioning Psychological functioning Social functioning Cognitive functioning	Parents and children 8–18 years old
Childhood Asthma Questionnaires[17]	Active quality of living Distress about asthma General health perceptions Positive quality of living	CAQ-A 4–7 years old (with parental help) CAQ-B 8–11 years old CAQ-C 12–16 years old

(Continued)

Table 5.1 Continued		
Questionnaire	Domains covered	Completed by
Impact of Childhood Illness Scale[24] (Epilepsy)	Impact on child Impact of epilepsy treatment Impact on family Impact on parents Cumulative impact Total Scale Scores	Parents of children 6–17 years old
Diabetes Quality of Life Measure[21]	Diabetes worries Disease impact Satisfaction of illness and treatment Social worries	Adolescents 13 years old and over

consist of three separate measures tailored to the developmental level and life context of three different age groups. The scale developed for the youngest age group (4–7 years old) contains 14 items that focus on emotions. Children respond on smiley face scales and complete the measure with parental help. The form for 8–11 year olds is longer (23 items), can be completed with help from an adult if required, and asks about frequencies of illness-related events as well as emotions. The form for 12–16 year contains 41 items, uses a numerical response scale, and is completed without assistance.

Who should complete the assessment?

Parental or caregiver assessments of health-related quality of life can supplement or be used as a proxy for the child assessments.

Carer assessments have been incorporated into some child quality of life measures to provide complementary information.[26,27] Insights into adjustment and development can be revealed because parent-rated quality of life is related to later adjustment of mothers and their children.[28] Similarly, carers can recognise the impact of the child's condition on the family.[29,30]

More fundamentally, the family is an important part of the child's environment; therefore his or her quality of life will be defined by family relationships.[31] At a more practical level carers both influence the health and provide care for children. Furthermore, chronic illness in a child is likely to affect the family and healthcare often seeks to help the parents as well as the child. Lastly, the impact of the child's condition on the family may influence a parent's appraisal of the child's condition.

This concern that the effect of a child's condition on a carer may influence the carer's assessment of the child's quality of life is one reason why the use of proxies might be avoided.[32]

The use of proxies to provide information about a child's quality of life presents some advantages. Parent-completed measures avoid the practical problems of reading level and comprehension. Parents, physicians, and teachers are indispensable sources of information about the quality of life of very young children or children who cannot complete these assessments.[19,24,33–35]

Unfortunately, only modest agreement is found between proxies and children's reports of quality of life.[36] Agreement is better between child and proxy reports of observable functioning than of non-observable emotional or social aspects,[37] which suggests the greater value of proxies' reports about more objective issues.

These low levels of agreement for non-observable domains reflect the proxies' limited knowledge about particular areas of the child's life. Health professionals have limited information about school, home life, and the subjective feelings of the child. Even parents have been found to have a poor perception of their children's problems and tend to report visible aspects of their child's condition compared to the subjective accounts given by children.[38,39]

Given these findings, it makes sense for children to complete quality of life assessments themselves wherever possible, especially as they have been found to provide reliable data.[40,41]

Implications for the future

The development of appropriate measures for children should be a priority. However, as there is little theoretical basis in existing scales for children's issues, new measures should be based on conceptual models tailored to the different stages of childhood.[42] Greater understanding of child quality of life could be achieved through more in-depth investigation of children's experiences through qualitative interviews and focus groups with children and parents as well as observational studies in schools. This would help ensure appropriate questionnaire content, types of question and response scales, and more effective administration methods.

In order to ensure that children understand quality of life assessments, separate measures and different administration methods should be adopted for the different age groups as demonstrated in the CHAQs.[17] The development of novel ways of administering quality of life questionnaires is also promising. In younger children, pictures, videos, story-telling techniques, and computer-aided administration of quality of life measures may increase comprehension as well as enjoyment of these assessments. This should also enhance completion of quality of life assessments and increase the accuracy of the information gathered.[43]

The use of proxy reports for the sake of convenience should be avoided.[44] However, developing parent and child versions of questionnaires would ensure that the quality of life of children who are not able to complete questionnaires is also assessed.[45] Proxy reports may also provide useful supplementary information, although further work is needed to determine the complementary roles of child and proxy completed scales.

The steps taken to improve child quality of life measures should advance understanding about the effects of illness in childhood. This should lead towards improvements in the education of health professionals working in this challenging field and in the provision of paediatric health care.

Box 5.2 Future research and education

Work should aim to:

- develop a consensual definition of quality of life in children
- investigate the effects of cognitive development and maturation upon perceptions of health and quality of life
- develop age-appropriate quality of life scales based on the experiences of children
- determine the complementary roles of proxy- and child-completed questionnaires
- educate health professionals about the effects of illness and treatment upon the physical and psychological development of children.

References

1. World Health Organization. *Constitution* Geneva: World Health Organization, 1946.
2. World Health Organization. *International classification of functioning, disability and health. Short version.* Geneva: World Health Organization, 2001.
3. Rosenbaum PL, Cadman D, Kirpalani H. Measuring health related quality of life in pediatric populations: conceptual issues. In: Spilker B, ed. *Quality of life assessments in clinical trials.* New York: Raven Press, 1990, pp. 205–15.
4. Allison PJ, Locker D, Feine, JS. Quality of life: a dynamic construct. *Soc Sci Med* 1997;**45**:221–30.
5. Titman P, Smith M, Graham P. Assessment of quality of life in children. *Clin Child Psychol Psychatr* 1997;**2**:597–606.
6. Spieth LE, Harris CV. Assessment of health-related quality of life in children and adolescents: an integrative review. *J Pediatr Psychol* 1995;**21**:175–93.
7. Millstein S, Irwin C. Concepts of health and illness: different constructs or variations on a theme. *Health Psychol* 1987; **6**:515–19.
8. Eiser C, Morse R. Quality of life measures in chronic diseases of childhood. *Health Technol Assess* 2001;**5**:1–157.
9. Nir M, Lanng S, Johanson HK, Koch, C. Long-term survival and nutritional data in patients with cystic fibrosis treated in a Danish centre. *Thorax* 1996;**51**:1023–7.
10. Roberts CS, Turney ME, Knowles AM. Psychosocial issues of adolescents with cancer. *Soc Work Health Care* 1998;**27**:3–18.

11. Feldman BM, Grundland B, McCullough, L, Wright V. Distinction of quality of life, health related quality of life, and health status in children referred for rheumatologic care. *J Rheumatol* 2000;**27**:226–33.

12. Feldman BM, Ayling-Campos A, Luy L *et al.* Measuring disability in juvenile dermatomyositis: validity of the childhood health assessment questionnaire. *J Rheumatol* 1995;**22**:326–31.

13. Berry SL, Hayford JR, Ross CK, Pachman LM, Lavigne JV. Conceptions of illness by children with juvenile rheumatoid arthritis: a cognitive developmental approach. *J Pediatr Psychol* 1993;**18**:83–97.

14. Juniper EF, Howland WC, Roberts NB, Thompson AK, King DR. Measuring quality of life in children with rhinoconjunctivitis. *J Allergy Clin Immunol* 1998;**101**:163–70.

15. Neff EJ, Dale JC. Assessment of quality of life in school-aged children: a method – phase 1. *Matern Child Nurs J* 1990;**19**:313–20.

16. Christie MJ, French D, Weatherstone L, West A, the Applied Psychology Research Group. The patients' perceptions of chronic disease and its management: psychosomatics, holism and quality of life in contemporary management of childhood asthma. *Psychother Psychosom* 1991;**56**:197–203.

17. Christie MJ, French D, Sowden A, West A. Development of child-centred disease specific questionnaires for living with asthma. *Psychosom Med* 1993;**55**:541–8.

18. Carr AJ, Gibson B, Robinson PG. Is quality of life determined by expectations or experience? *BMJ* 2001;**322**:1240–43.

19. Hanai T. Quality of life in children with epilepsy. *Epilepsia* 1996;**37**:28–33.

20. Pal DK. Quality of life assessment in children: a review of conceptual and methodological issues in multidimensional health status measures. *J Epidemiol Community Health* 1996;**50**:391–6.

21. Diabetes Control and Complications Trial (DCCT) Research Group. Reliability and validity of a diabetes quality of life measure for The Diabetes Control and Complications Trial (DCCT). *Diabetes Care* 1988;**11**:725–32.

22. Kaplan RM, Bush JW, Berry CC. Health states: types of validity and the index of well-being. *Health Serv Res* 1976;**11**:478–507.

23. Varni JW, Katz ER, Seid M, Quiggins DJL, Friedman-Bender A. The Pediatric Cancer Quality of Life Inventory-32 (PCQL-32) 1. Reliability and validity. *Cancer* 1998;**82**:1184–96.

24. Hoare P, Russell M. The quality of life of children with chronic epilepsy and their families: Preliminary findings with a new assessment measure. *Dev Med Child Neurol* 1995;**37**:689–96.

25. Starfield B, Bergner M, Ensminger M *et al*. Adolescent health status measurement: development of the Child Health and Illness Profile. *Pediatr* 1993;**91**:430–35.

26. Stein R, Riessman C. The development of the Impact-on-Family Scale: preliminary findings. *Med Care* 1980;**18**:465–72.

27. Juniper EF, Guyatt GH, Feeny D *et al*. Measuring quality of life in parents of children with asthma. *Qual Life Res* 1996;**5**:27–36.

28. Kazak AE, Barakat LP. Brief report: parenting stress and quality of life during treatment for childhood leukemia predicts child and parent adjustment after treatment ends. *J Pediatr Psychol* 1997;**22**:749–58.

29. Rothman ML, Hendrick SC, Blucroft KA, Hickman DH, Rubenstein LZ. The validity of proxy generated scores as measures of patient health status. *Med Care* 1991;**29**:115–24.

30. Hanson CL. Quality of life in families of youths with chronic conditions. In: Koot HM, Wallander JL, eds. *Quality of life in child and adolescent illness*. Hove: Brunner-Routledge, 2001, pp. 181–209.

31. Fink R. Issues and problems in measuring children's health status in community health research. *Soc Sci Med* 1989;**29**: 715–19.

32. Osman L, Silverman M. Measuring quality of life for young children with asthma and their families. *Eur Respir J* 1996; **9**(suppl 21):35–41.

33. Goodwin DAJ, Boggs SR, Graham-Pole J. Development and validation of the Pediatric Oncology Quality of Life Scale. *Psychol Assess* 1994;**6**:321–8.

34. Feeny D, Furlong W, Barr RD *et al*. A comprehensive multiattribute system for classifying the health status of survivors of childhood cancer. *J Clin Oncol* 1992;**10**:923–8.

35. Finkelstein JW. Methods, models, and measures of health-related quality of life for children and adolescents. In: Drotar D, ed. *Measuring health-related quality of life in children and adolescents. Implications for research and practice*. New Jersey: Lawrence Erlbaum Associates Inc., 1998, pp. 39–52.

36. Achenbach TM, McConaughy SH, Howell CT. Child/adolescent behavioural and emotional problems: implications of cross-informant correlations for situational specificity. *Psychol Bull* 1987;**101**:213–32.

37. Eiser C, Morse R. Can parents rate their child's health-related quality of life? *Qual Life Res* 2001;**10**:347–57.

38. Juniper EF, Guyatt GH, Dolovich, J. Assessment of quality of life in adolescents with allergic rhinoconjunctivitis: development and testing of a questionnaire for clinical trials. *J Allergy Clin Immunol* 1993;**93**:413–21.

39. Kazdin AE, French NH, Unis AS. Child, mother and father evaluations of depression in psychiatric inpatient children. *J Abnorm Child Psychol* 1983;**11**:167–80.

40. Feeny D, Juniper EF, Ferrie PJ, Griffith LE, Guyatt GH. Why not just ask the kids? Health-related quality of life in children with asthma. In: Drotar D, ed. *Measuring health-related quality of life in children and adolescents. Implications for research and practice.* New Jersey: Lawrence Erlbaum Associates Inc., 1998, pp. 171–85.

41. French DJ, Christie MJ, Sowden AJ. The reproducibility of the childhood asthma questionnaires: measures of quality of life for children with asthma 4–16 years. *Qual Life Res* 1994;**3**:215–24.

42. Wilson IB, Cleary PD. Linking clinical variables with health-related quality of life. *JAMA* 1995;**273**:59–65.

43. Jenney MEM, Campbell S. Measuring quality of life. *Arch Dis Child* 1997;**77**:347–50.

44. Cella DF, Tulsky DS. Quality of life in cancer: definition, purpose and method of measurement. *Cancer Invest* 1993;**11**:327–36.

45. Landgraf JM, Maunsell KNS, Bullinger M *et al*. Canadian, French, German and UK versions of the Child Health Questionnaire: ethodology and preliminary item scaling results. *Qual Life Res* 1998;**7**:433–45.

6: Who should measure quality of life?

JULIA ADDINGTON-HALL AND LALIT KALRA

Summary points

- Some patients cannot complete quality of life measures because they have cognitive impairments, communication deficits, are in severe distress or because the measures are too burdensome.
- It is precisely these patients for whom information on quality of life is most needed to inform decision-making.
- Proxies – both healthcare professionals and lay caregivers – can provide useful information, particularly on the more concrete, observable aspects of quality of life.
- Scores from proxies may be influenced by their own feelings about and experiences of caring for the patient.
- Clinicians should remember that when their assessment of quality of life is at odds with that of the patient, it is the patient who should have the final word.

Introduction

One of the reasons behind the rapid development of quality of life measures in healthcare has been the growing recognition of the importance of understanding the impact of healthcare interventions on patients' lives, rather than just on their bodies. This is particularly important for patients with chronic, disabling, or life-threatening diseases, who live without the expectation of cure and with conditions that are likely to impact on their physical, psychological, and social wellbeing. Health professionals frequently resort to quality of life judgements, even ahead of survival, in the management of disabled patients,[1] and the professional view on expected quality of life is often the key factor in effective treatment for a life-threatening condition not being given or being withdrawn.[2] Their perceptions may, however, be at odds with those held by patients.[3] It is therefore important to ask patients to assess their own quality of life, using one of a growing number of reliable and valid measures. Choosing an appropriate measure and using it in clinical practice can be problematic,[4] as discussed in Chapter 3. This presupposes, however, that patients are able to assess their own quality of life and to complete a quality of life measure. Some – and in some conditions, many – patients are unable to do this because of cognitive impairments, communications deficits, severe symptom distress, or because the quality of life measure is physically or emotionally too burdensome.[5] These may be precisely the patients for whom information on quality of life is most needed to inform clinical decision-making. Rather than lose all information on that patient, someone else (a family member or health professional) may be asked to act as a proxy or surrogate. The issue in quality of life measurement addressed in this paper is the use of proxies to measure quality of life. We will consider the advantages and disadvantages of using proxies to rate quality of life, debate the reasons why proxy and patient views may differ, and suggest directions for future research.

Can proxies provide useful information on quality of life?

Quality of life tools measure subjective experience. Completing a quality of life measure on behalf of someone else therefore requires the proxy to put themselves in the other person's shoes, to imagine what it feels like to be them, and to speculate about the impact of their health and healthcare on their experience of life. Proxies are often rather good at this. There is usually moderate agreement between individual patients and their proxies, although lower levels of agreement may be reported for psychosocial functioning.[5,6] For example, cancer patients' ratings of seven domains of quality of life (physical fitness, feelings, daily and social activities, overall health, pain, and overall quality of life) on a five-point scale agreed exactly with those of their "significant other" (usually a spouse), agreed with doctors and nurses on 41% of all comparisons made, and were within one response category for 43% of comparisons with only 17% showing more profound discrepancies.[7] Proxies are almost as good as patients in detecting changes in some quality of life domains over time.[8] At a group level, there is a tendency for proxies to rate quality of life as more impaired than the patient.[5] This depends, however, both on the domain and on the type of proxy. Nurses[6] and lay caregivers[9] are particularly likely to overestimate the patients' levels of depression, anxiety, and distress, whilst a number of studies have shown that doctors consistently underestimate the severity of symptoms.[10,11] Although proxy and patient ratings do not agree exactly, there appears to be sufficient agreement between patients' and proxies' quality of life assessments to make the information they provide useful in situations when the patient cannot be asked directly.[6]

A number of factors have been identified that affect the degree of agreement between patients and proxies. These are reviewed in Table 6.1. Although it is important to be aware that patient and proxy characteristics can affect agreement, they have small effects. For example, patient and proxy characteristics accounted for less than 15% of the variance in patient-proxy differences in a study comparing cancer patient and proxy scores on the European Organisation for Research and Treatment into Cancer (EORTC QLQ-30).[5] This may suggest that important determinants of the agreement between proxy and patient ratings have yet to be identified. Whilst more research is needed to investigate this, the authors argue that it is more likely that random error in both patient and proxy ratings accounts for most of the difference between the two from, for example, a lack of precision in the tools used and situational factors such as mood.

Further understanding of why proxy and patient scores on quality of life measures differ may come from a greater understanding of the determinants of an individual's assessments of quality of life. These are considered in the next section.

Table 6.1 Factors affecting agreement in quality of life assessments

General factors	Factors related to the patient	Factors related to the proxy
Agreement depends on the concreteness, visibility, and importance of the aspects of quality of life under consideration.[6] Agreement is better for concrete, observable aspects and less good for more subjective domains, such as emotional health	Patients may not complete quality of life measures in ways that accurately reflect their feelings. For example, patients may seek to answer questions in ways that present themselves favourably. This may be related to findings of lesser agreement between patients and proxies[4]	The lay caregivers' experience of caring, the amount of time they spend with the patient, and their own distress may influence their assessment of the patient's quality of life.
Agreement may improve over time, but evidence is contradictory	Proxies have a better chance of accurately reflecting quality of life if patients are open with them about their problems and feelings	Lower quality of life scores have been associated with increases in the burden on the caregiver,[24,25] time spent together,[26] and the carer's distress,[13] and with the carer having a lower quality of life[5]
The psychometric properties of the measure are important: if the measure is unreliable, then high agreement cannot be expected	Agreement between patients and proxies seems to be greater when quality of life is either very good or very poor	Extent of agreement may be influenced by the relationship between the patient and proxy, although the evidence for this is limited
		Health professionals may project their own feelings of hopelessness and distress on to the patient when assessing their quality of life[27,28]

Determinants of quality of life scores

There is no direct correspondence between objective functioning and the individual's quality of life nor between the perceptions of patients and healthy people, professionals or even others with similar disabilities.[12-14] Patients may rate their quality of life highly despite obvious problems or may show significant improvement in quality of life scores that do not correlate with objective measures of disease activity or physical function. Clinicians may find it difficult to believe patients' ratings of quality of life. This can be a particular issue when working with patients with severe disabilities or with those at the end of life, where clinicians may hold expectations about quality of life that are not supported by patient's self-assessments.

It is, for example, often presumed that dying is a time of great suffering and severe problems,[15] and that quality of life scores will therefore decline as death approaches. Indeed, in a study comparing quality of life measures in advanced cancer patients it was argued that the fact that one measure showed greater deterioration over time than another suggested that this measure was more sensitive.[16] The functional status of cancer patients does decline as death approaches and is a good prognostic indicator.[17] Scores on other quality of life domains are neither necessarily lower than in other people nor necessarily deteriorate. For example, hospice patients had lower scores than apparently healthy adults on two quality of life domains (psychophysiological wellbeing and functional wellbeing) but not on a third (social and spiritual wellbeing).[18] The implications of this "disability paradox" for comparative quality of life measurement using methods such as quality adjusted life years is discussed elsewhere.[4] Patients' priorities may change at the end of life. It has been argued that existential, spiritual, and social issues become more important.[19] For example, in a study using an individualised quality of life measure, SEIQoL, with patients with advanced incurable cancer, family concerns were almost universally rated as more important than health in determining quality of life.[20] Of a possible score of 100, the median global quality of life score was 61, challenging the belief that terminally ill patients invariably have poor quality of life.

It has been argued that changes in quality of life in chronic and life-threatening illnesses result in part from adaptation to the situation in which the patient finds him or herself[21] (Box 6.1). Patients change their internal standards, values and/or conceptualisation of quality of life and therefore assess it differently from the way they would have done if they had not adapted to their situation. This phenomenon of internal adaptation is called "response shift" and may explain apparently paradoxical quality of life scores in these patients. It is demonstrated in reverse by the finding that pre-transplantation kidney patients' mean rating of quality of life was 5·23 on a ten-point scale, which rose to 7 after transplantation.[22] When asked to rate their quality of life before transplantation five, 12 and 18 months after successful transplantation they retrospectively gave it scores of 3·27, 3·14 and 3·05. Patients had successfully adapted to their condition before treatment, and thus rated their quality of life more highly than they did when they re-evaluated it from the vantage point of improved health after the operation. It has been noted above that proxies tend to rate patients' quality of life as being worse than patients think it is. Response shift may account for this.

Box 6.1 Determinants of changes in self assessment of quality of life[21]

According to a theoretical model developed by Sprangers and Schwartz,[21] changes may result from an interaction between:

- a catalyst, such as a change in health status
- antecedents – that is, stable characteristics or the individual's disposition, for example personality traits
- mechanisms – that is, behavioural, cognitive, and affective processes that accommodate changes in health status, for example comparing oneself to others, adjusting goals, adopting different routines
- response shift – that is, "changes in the meaning of one's evaluation of quality of life resulting from changes in internal standards, values, or conceptualisation".[21]

Response shift has received little attention until recently but it has important implications for measurement of change in quality of life. Greater understanding of how patient and proxy evaluations of quality of life change over time would help to explain why proxy and patient ratings do not always agree and might help us to interpret changes in quality of life scores more meaningfully. Some of the problems posed by response shift in measuring change in quality of life were highlighted in Chapter 2.[23]

Discussion and future issues

Quality of life measures are designed to enable the patients' perspective on the impact of health and healthcare interventions on their lives to be assessed and taken into account in clinical decision-making and research. Some patients are unable to complete these measures due to cognitive impairments, communication deficits, severe distress, or because these measures are too burdensome for them. It is precisely these patients, however, where information on quality of life is most needed to inform decision-making. The evidence on using proxies to measure quality of life suggests that both healthcare professionals and lay caregivers can provide useful information, particularly on more concrete, observable aspects of quality of life. Proxies' scores may be influenced by their own feelings and experiences when caring for the patient, and the extent to which patients normally talk about their feelings seems important. It is likely that agreement will be greater when reliable measures are used, although this has not been empirically tested. Further research is needed to understand fully how the characteristics of patient, proxy, and measure influence agreement. In particular, greater understanding is needed of how expectations and adaptation influence individuals' assessments of their quality of life. In the meantime, clinicians would do well to remember that when their assessment of quality of life is at odds with that of the patient, it is the patient who should have the final word.

Acknowledgements

We thank our colleagues in the Interdisciplinary Research Group in Palliative and Person Centred Care at King's College London, in particular Irene Higginson, Peter Robinson,

Alison Carr, Barry Gibson, Stanley Gelbier, Robert Dunlop and Alan Turner-Smith, who have participated in discussions and commented on an earlier draft of this work.

References

1. Manara AR, Pittman JA, Braddon FE. Reasons for withdrawing treatment in patients receiving intensive care. *Anaesth* 1998; 53:523–8.
2. Pellegrino ED. Decisions to withdraw life-sustaining treatment: a moral algorithm. *JAMA* 2000;**283**:1065–7.
3. Hallan S, Asberg A, Indredavik B, Wideroe TE. Quality of life after cerebrovascular stroke: a systematic study of patients' preferences for different functional outcomes. *J Intern Med* 1999; **246**:309–16.
4. Higginson IJ, Carr AJ. How can quality of life measures be used in the clinical setting? *BMJ* 2001;**322**:1297–1300.
5. Sneeuw KC, Aaronson NK, Sprangers MA *et al*. EORTC QLQ-C30 ratings in assessing the quality of life of cancer patients. *J Clin Epidemiol* 1998;**51**:617–31.
6. Sprangers MAG, Aaronson NK. The role of health care providers and significant others in evaluating the quality of life of patients with chronic disease: a review. *J Clin Epidemiol* 1992;**45**:743–60.
7. Sneeuw KC, Aaronson NK, Sprangers MA *et al*. Evaluating the quality of life of cancer patients: assessments by patients, significant others, physicians and nurses. *Br J Cancer* 1999;**81**: 87–94.
8. Sneeuw KCA, Aaronson NK, Sprangers MA *et al*. Value of caregiver ratings in evaluating the quality of life of patients with cancer. *J Clin Oncol* 1997;**15**:1206–17.
9. Spiller JA. Alexander DA. Domiciliary care: a comparison of the views of terminally ill patients and their family caregivers. *Palliative Med* 1993;**7**:109–15.
10. Stephens RJ, Hopwood P, Girling DJ, Machin D. Randomised trials with quality of life endpoints: are doctors' ratings of patients' physical symptoms interchangeable with patients' self-ratings? *Qual Life Res* 1997;**6**:225–36.
11. Nekolaichuk CL, Bruera E, Spachynski K, MacEachern T. A comparison of patient and proxy symptom assessments in advanced cancer patients. *Palliative Med* 1999;**13**:311–23.
12. Rothwell PM, McDowell Z, Wong CK, Dorman PJ. Doctors and patients don't agree: cross sectional study of patients' and doctors' perceptions and assessments of disability in multiple sclerosis. *BMJ* 1997;**314**:1580–83.

13. Pierre U, Wood-Dauphinee S, Korner-Bitensky N, Gayton D, Hanley J. Proxy use of the Canadian SF-36 in rating health status of the disabled elderly. *J Clin Epidemiol* 1998;**51**:983–90.

14. Ebrahim S, Brittis S, Wu A. The valuation of states of ill-health: the impact of age and disability. *Age Ageing* 1991;**20**:37–40.

15. Stewart AL, Teno J, Patrick DL, Lynn J. The concept of quality of life of dying persons in the context of health care. *J Pain Symptom Manage* 1999;**17**:93–108.

16. Sloan JA, Loprinzi CL, Kuross SA *et al.* Randomised comparison of four tools measuring overall quality of life in patients with advanced cancer. *J Clin Oncol* 1998;**16**:3662–73.

17. Vigano A, Dorgan M, Buckingham J, Bruera E, Suarez-Almazor ME. Survival prediction in terminal cancer patients: a systematic review of the medical literature. *Palliative Med* 2000;**14**:363–74.

18. McMillan SC, Weitzner M. Quality of life in cancer patients: use of a revised Hospice Index. *Cancer Pract* 1999;**6**:282–8.

19. Cohen R, Mount BM. Quality of life in terminal illness: defining and measuring subjective well-being in the dying. *J Palliative Care* 1992;**8**:40–45.

20. Waldron D, O'Boyle CA, Kearney M, Moriarty M, Carney D. Quality of life measurement in advanced cancer: assessing the individual. *J Clin Oncol* 1999;**17**:3603–11.

21. Sprangers MA, Schwartz CE. Integrating response shift into health-related quality of life research: a theoretical model. *Soc Sci Med* 1999;**48**:1507–15.

22. Adang EMM, Kootstra G, van Hoeff JP, Merckelbach HLGJ. Do retrospective and prospective quality of life assessments differ for pancreas–kidney transplant recipients? *Transplant Int* 1998;**11**:11–15.

23. Carr AJ, Gibson BA, Robinson PG. Is quality of life determined by expectations or experience? *BMJ* 2001;**322**:1240–43.

24. Rothman ML, Hedrick SC, Bulcroft KA, Hickman DH, Rubenstein LZ. The validity of proxy-generated scores as measures of patient health status. *Med Care* 1991;**29**:115–24.

25. Clipp EC, George LK. Patients with cancer and their spouse caregivers: perceptions of the illness experience. *Cancer* 1992;**69**:1074–9.

26. Epstein AM, Hall JA, Tognetti J, Son LH, Conant L. Using proxies to evaluate quality of life. *Med Care* 1989;**27**(suppl 3):91–8.

27. Husted SA, Johnson JG. Oncology clients' affective states and their nurses' expectations of clients' affective states. *Cancer Nurs* 1985;**8**:159–65.

28. Jennings BM, Muhlenkamp AF. Systematic misperception: oncology patients' self-reported affective states and their caregivers' perceptions. *Cancer Nurs* 1981;**4**:485–9.

7: The clinical utility of quality of life measures

IRENE J HIGGINSON AND ALISON J CARR

Summary points

- Quality of life measures can provide a means of capturing the personal and social context of care.
- These have potential uses in both the clinical encounter (prioritising problems, communication, screening for potential problems, identifying preferences, monitoring change or response to treatment) and in quality improvement (training new staff, clinical audit, and clinical governance).
- Quality of life measures are not a substitute for disease outcomes and may not always be the most appropriate patient-centred outcome to assess. The choice of outcome measure will depend upon the purpose of treatment and evaluation.
- There are ethical considerations in the use of quality of life measures. They may raise expectations that treatment will be able to solve problems that are outside the remit of healthcare.
- Measures developed for research often do not easily transfer to clinical practice – either because they are too long for routine use or because they fail to capture clinical important aspects of care and changes.
- Measures designed specifically for clinical care are being developed.
- Measures that form an integral part of treatment planning and evaluation are more likely to influence clinical decision making than those that are simply used to monitor disease or treatment.

Introduction

In modern medicine the traditional way of assessing change among patients has been to focus on laboratory or clinical tests. At its most simple, this involves measuring pulse, blood pressure, temperature, and carrying out physical examinations. At the more complex, it includes haematological analysis, CT scans, radiographs, organ function tests, genetic analysis, and many other investigations. Whilst these give important information about the disease, in chronic and progressive disease in particular, it is impossible to separate the disease from the individual's personal and social context. No illness exists in a vacuum.

One way of capturing the personal and social context of patients is to use quality of life measures.[1] These are accepted outcome measures in clinical research but are rarely used in routine clinical practice, despite the fact that Florence Nightingale was one of the first clinicians to insist on measuring the outcome of routine care, to evaluate treatment.[2] This chapter reviews the particular challenges of using quality of life measures in clinical practice. Selection of appropriate measures, analysis of quality of life data, feedback and interpretation of results in practice, and incorporation into clinical decision-making will be discussed. The chapter will examine practical ways of resolving the tension between the need for approaches suitable in the clinical encounter and the highly individualised nature of quality of life.

Use of quality of life measures in clinical practice

Quality of life measures have eight potential uses to aid routine clinical practice:

- prioritising problems
- communication
- screening for potential problems
- identifying preferences
- monitoring change or response to treatment
- training new staff
- in clinical audit
- and in clinical governance (see Tables 7.1 and 7.2).

The first five of these can be of immediate value in the clinical encounter, while the last three contribute to training, review of care, and its improvement in the future.

Table 7.1 Use of quality of life measures in the clinical encounter

Potential use of quality of life measures in routine practice	Examples of application
Identifying and prioritising problems	By recording information on a range of problems the patient and the doctor or nurse can discuss and identify which appears to be most important problem and thus agree that this is the priority for action. This is particularly useful when patients have multiple problems, for example in the elderly or in those receiving palliative care.[3] In addition, quality of life measures can be used to capture information that appears superficially to have no clinical relevance but which can explain disease severity or coping problems.[4]
Communication: (1) from patient to doctors and nurses (2) between health staff and (3) between the patient and his/her family or friends	A patient-completed quality of life assessment can help patients to convey their problems to doctors, nurses or other staff because it quickly presents information on the patient's assessment of a range of problems. If correctly applied it may speed up the clinical encounter, and help to focus on the patient's main concerns.
Screening for hidden problems or use as a checklist to alert clinicians of aspects of care they may have overlooked	Some patient's problems can be overlooked unless specifically enquired about. These particularly include psychological and social problems.[5] For example, a measure that asks the question: "would you describe your mood as depressed most of the time?" is a sensitive and specific screening tool for depression. These aspects may have an important effect on treatment or care.
Identifying patient preferences to facilitate shared clinical decision-making	These help to identify the patient's preferred outcome or goals of treatment. If these are not known, then the treatment prescribed may not meet the patient's preference and this may in turn affect adherence to treatment and patient satisfaction.
Monitoring changes or response to treatment in an individual	At the moment change is largely monitored through laboratory or clinical tests, rather than the patient's perception of change. Inability to bring about improvements that are seen as relevant to the patient may affect adherence to treatment.

Table 7.2 Use of quality of life measures in quality improvement

Potential use of quality of life measure in routine practice	Examples of application
Training new staff in assessment	Training doctors and nurses has moved away from a purely knowledge-based system to encompass training in skills. However, staff can often overlook aspects of care, especially those relating to quality of life. Quality of life measures that include a breakdown of aspects important to the person (such as symptoms, functioning, and psychological and social wellbeing) can enable the new clinician to gain an overview of the person's problems. It can also help to prioritise when there are several difficulties. Training can include clinical assessment and interviewing skills[6] along with the use of quality of life measures.
Clinical audit	Quality of life measures are an important part of the systematic assessment of the outcomes or results of care. Review of aspects of care that are and are not achieved, or of those individual patients where outcomes were not achieved as wished can help staff to prepare plans to deal better with those problems in the future. For example, this has included: training staff to manage the problem more effectively,[7] change in organisational aspects of care or development of predictive information to identify, at an earlier stage, those patients with problems.[8] Including quality of life measures in clinical audit ensures that the audit concentrates on what is important to patients, rather than technical aspects of quality.
Clinical governances	Quality of life measures can be incorporated in the framework of continual improvement and review encouraged by the new guidance on clinical governance. Assessing the quality of life of patients ensures that clinical governance focuses on what is important to patients and their families. Along with mortality and satisfaction, it is increasingly used as a criterion by which services and treatments are evaluated.

Pitfalls and problems with quality of life measures in clinical practice

The underlying reason for using quality of life measures in clinical practice is to ensure that treatment plans and evaluations are centred on the patient rather than the disease. Quality of life is not the only way to capture patient-centred outcomes; measures of disability, social interaction and support, and of psychological wellbeing can be appropriate. Quality of life measures are not a substitute for disease outcomes but an adjunct to them: for example, rheumatologists would not treat rheumatoid arthritis with disease-modifying anti-rheumatic drugs simply on the basis of quality of life scores. Similarly, broad, multidimensional quality of life measures may be less effective, accurate, and responsive than measures of specific patient outcomes (for example, anxiety and depression) in situations where treatment is aimed at that outcome. Quality of life is a highly individual concept: Mount and Scott likened assessing it to assessing the beauty of a rose.[9] No matter how many measurements are made (for example, of colour, smell, and height), the full beauty of the rose is never captured. Quality of life measures will never capture all aspects important to an individual, although systems where patients generate at least some of the aspects are likely to be closest. The individual nature and the shortcomings of many existing quality of life measures are discussed further in Chapter 3.

Routine use of quality of life measures is no substitute for proper training of staff. There is a potential danger that staff may see the use of the assessment as an alternative to communicating with patients, rather than as an aid to care. However, it is also important to train staff in the use of quality of life measures – something generally lacking in current undergraduate and postgraduate training. In clinical governance and audit, caution is needed when interpreting the results of quality of life assessments, and any other outcome measure, among patients with different case-mix.

Ethical considerations

The breadth of quality of life as a concept means that problems might be identified that are outside the usual remit of medical care.[10] This raises a number of ethical concerns. First, the act of measuring quality of life in a clinical setting may generate the expectation that the clinician will be able to influence it; otherwise, what would be the purpose of measuring it? In situations where this is not possible, patients may be seen to be harmed by the process of measurement. Second, some pressure groups such as the Movement for Independent Living have opposed clinical measurement of quality of life on the grounds that it represents "overmedicalisation"; clinical interference in aspects of patients' lives that should not be the concern of the clinician. On the other hand, data from quality of life measures could be used to lobby for deficient resources or to inform health and social policy. Finally, chronic disease affects and is affected by the broader aspects of people's lives such as their relationships and social support, and such information can influence treatment decisions and assessments of healthcare need.

Considerations when measuring quality of life in clinical practice

Properties of the measure

In addition to the properties needed when using a measure in research, such as validity and reliability, in clinical practice a wider range of properties is required to ensure the measure is feasible for routine use. These properties include the appropriateness and acceptability of the measure, its responsiveness to clinical change, and its interpretability (Box 7.1).

Box 7.1 Properties required of measures used in clinical practice

Validity assesses whether the instrument measures what you intend to measure, i.e. quality of life. There are several questions to be considered when assessing the validity of measures for clinical practice.

- Does the measure cover aspects that are clinically relevant to patients, their families and to professionals? (face validity)

- Are the domains appropriate, important and sufficient for the setting or types of patients being studied? (content validity)
- Does the measure correlate with a gold standard or superior measure? (criterion validity). If this is not known, because there is no gold standard, then an alternative question is whether the measure produces results that conform to a theory. For example, a measure of weakness correlates with a patient's stage of disease. This test, however, is only as good as the theory used.

Appropriateness and acceptability assess whether the measure is suitable for its intended use. This is crucial in clinical practice, where measures must be simple to use. There are several questions to be answered.

- Is the measure short/long enough for completion or administration in the intended setting and with the types of patients, families or informants?
- Are the format of the measure and questions acceptable and suitable for administration in the intended setting and with the intended informants?
- Has it been used in this or similar settings before, and did it work?
- If the measure is a translation, will it work in this culture and language? Has there been a double translation? Has its conceptual as well as its semantic equivalence been assessed?

Reliability assesses whether the measure produces the same results when repeated in an unchanged population. This includes the inter-rater (or interobserver) reliability, which tests for similar results with different observers, and the test–retest reliability, which tests for similar results when used at different points in time. Another test sometimes used is whether individual items of the measure correlate with each other (this is called internal consistency). This is not a true test of reliability. If a measure has a very high internal consistency, although it is likely that the measure is reliable, it also suggests that many items in the measure are capturing the same things. Thus, some may be redundant and the measure could be shortened.

Responsiveness to change is whether the measure can detect clinically meaningful changes. This is sometimes called sensitivity. This is critical if the measure is to be of any use in clinical practice. For example, will the measure discriminate between different degrees of severity, or detect changes anticipated by the treatment proposed? Among patients who have a progressive or advanced illness, many quality of life measures indicate poor scores (so-called floor effects), because they rely heavily on function as part of the quality of life assessment. Thus, changes in symptoms, family support or other important components of care are not detected.

Interpretability is whether the results from using the measure have clinical interpretation and relevance. When given a quality of life score, or a series of quality of life scores over time, the clinician needs to be able to consider what to do with this information. For example, an overall quality of life score – of say 5 out of 10 – offers little help when planning treatment. The clinician needs to understand what aspects are impeding quality of life – for example, symptoms, informational concerns, worries, etc. so that treatment can be planned. To be clinically useful measures must be able to provide easy access to the components of the assessment.

Transferability of measures from research to clinical practice

Identified barriers to the routine clinical use of outcome measures such as quality of life include concerns about cost, feasibility, and clinical relevance.[11] For a measure to have clinical utility it must possess all the properties listed above but must also be simple, quick to complete, easy to score, and provide data that are immediately and obviously clinically interpretable.[12] Most existing measures were developed for use in clinical research[13] where time and budgetary constraints are different from those in clinical practice. Some quality of life measures require trained staff to administer them and are time-consuming, taking 20 to 30 minutes to complete. Similarly, since the purpose of quality of life measurement in clinical trials is to compare groups of patients (usually over relatively short time periods), assessment of existing measures has focused on their performance in these situations. Such situations are very different from clinical practice where the purpose of measurement is to assess change in individual patients, in some instances over many years.[14] Furthermore, quality of life measures that quantify the broader context of patients' lives are likely to be influenced by events occurring throughout the patient's life course and it is not yet clear how changes in these measures should be interpreted over long periods of time. This is the problem of "response shift" that was discussed in chapters 2 and 6.

A small but growing number of quality of life instruments developed specifically for use in clinical practice are available.

One example of this is the Disease Repercussion Profile,[15] which assesses patient-perceived handicap in rheumatoid arthritis, osteoarthritis, and back pain. Other examples include the Support Team Assessment Schedule,[16] the Edmonton Symptom Assessment Scale,[17] and the Palliative Outcome Scale,[18] which were all developed specifically for palliative practice, and MYMOP,[19] which was designed for use in primary care. The properties of many of these instruments have been established but trials of their use in clinical practice are required to evaluate their routine use in this context.

Interpretation of results: mean score or severe score?

In research studies, quality of life measures are often presented using mean scores.[20] While this is useful in testing one treatment against another in groups of patients, it is of less value in clinical practice. At what point is a problem considered to be severe? Is it above the mean? Or a top quartile of scores? The decision here is clinical. Some screening scales have cut-off points for clinical intervention (for example, depression scales), but for others, whether the problem is rated as severe is more important.[18] Reducing the number of patients with severe pain was considered to be the clinically important aspect of one assessment scale.

Introduction and review: a practical guide

Introducing quality of life measures into clinical practice often means a change in practice for staff. Change can be threatening, especially if staff perceive that they may be judged adversely as a result. The organisation's culture becomes important.[21] As for any new assessment, staff need training in its use and interpretation. To be of most value quality of life measures should be incorporated into the clinical record, and the results discussed at clinical review meetings.[22] Suggested steps for choosing and introducing a quality of life measure into clinical practice are shown in Boxes 7.2 and 7.3.

Box 7.2 Ten steps for assessing and choosing a quality of life measure for clinical practice

1 Are the domains covered relevant?
2 What population and setting was it developed and tested in and are these similar to those planned for use?
3 What is the validity, reliability, responsiveness, and appropriateness of the measure?
4 What were the assumptions of the assessors when determining validity?
5 Are there floor and ceiling effects?
6 Will it measure differences between patients or over time – and at what power?
7 Who completes the measure? Patient, family, professional (and what effect will this have, will they be willing to complete it)?
8 How long does the measure take to complete?
9 Do staff and patients consider it easy to use?
10 Who requires training and information about the measure?

Box 7.3 Introducing a quality of life measure into clinical practice

- Review who else is doing what
- Make the initial choice
- Decide whether other outcomes also need to be monitored
- Get staff and patients involved
- Adapt for local use and own requirements
- Identify a leader of the project
- Assign responsibilities – who will be doing what
- Agree a timetable
- Test when and where the measure will be completed
- Prepare and test paperwork
- Plan and begin training both in the use of the quality of life measure and in associated clinical skills (this can be part of general staff training – for example, in communication and assessment)
- Agree start date and review period
- Begin to use the measure
- Review its use in the first week, first month, and then at regular intervals
- Review results of individual patients and groups to improve care
- Modify as patients and staff feel appropriate to improve the use of the measure, or make other changes

Does using quality of life measures improve care?

The individual patient

The potential benefit to the patient of using quality of life measures in clinical practice is that his/her problems are identified and dealt with and that treatment decisions are based on his/her priorities and preferences. Evidence for these benefits is lacking because quality of life measures are still rarely used in clinical practice. In rheumatology, where quality of life has been an important outcome in clinical trials for 15 to 20 years, surveys in the UK suggest that little use is made of quality of life measures in clinical practice.[23] Moreover, there is some suggestion that even where quality of life measures are used, they do not influence clinical decision-making. Clinical judgement analysis has highlighted discrepancies between the ways some clinicians think they make clinical decisions, and the weights they actually apply in practice.[24] The effect of information from quality of life measures on clinical decision-making appears small[25] but these data were collected before the introduction of high profile quality of life measures (such as the SF-36). One way of ensuring that quality of life assessments influence clinical decision-making is to use them as a basis for treatment choices. This can be effected by using quality of life measures to identify individual patients' problems and priorities for treatment and then negotiating treatment goals based on those priorities and preferences. An evaluation of the role of quality of life measures in clinical goal-setting is in progress.

The clinical service

There is often a lack of evidence to demonstrate that findings from audit or similar initiatives have resulted in a change in practice. Simply realising that a problem exists does not indicate what exactly needs to be changed in the clinical service.[26] Evaluation of audits in one health region identified changes in clinical services in the development and implementation of new standards of care, improvements in documentation, and specific clinical practice changes, such as prescribing, management of accidents, and seeking information.[27] However, there was no analysis of whether patient outcomes changed, and further work is needed to assess this. Using quality of life measures, such as QALYs (Quality Adjusted Life Years) to determine the relative value of different services or interventions is made difficult by the existence of the "disability paradox". People with important, even life threatening disease may not rate their quality of life as significantly poorer than people with mild disease or poorer than a healthy population. This makes direct comparisons between different disease groups for the purposes of resource allocation difficult.

Discussion and future directions

Technology

Many of the practical problems associated with quality of life measurement in clinical practice may be overcome by the use of new technologies. Computerised approaches to data storage and retrieval will simplify the collection, storage, and monitoring of quality of life data. The administration of quality of life measures via the internet, on touch-screen or palm top computers will overcome some of the problems of questionnaire administration and scoring. Data can be automatically downloaded to individual patient records where they can be reviewed in the context of their current treatment and clinical outcomes.

Individualised measures

The increasing interest in individualised quality of life measures reflects a perception that quality of life is unique to individuals and cannot be adequately assessed by standardised measures that ask all patients the same question and require them to choose from a set of pre-determined responses. The extent to which existing quality of life measures capture the quality of life of individual patients is discussed in Chapter 3. Individualised measures such as the Schedule for the Evaluation of Individualised Quality of Life (SEIQoL)[28] and the

Patient Generated Index (PGI),[29] ask the same question of each patient but allow individual patients to specify their own responses. Whilst the use of individualised measures of quality of life in research has been limited by difficulties in administration and scoring, in clinical practice they have immediate relevance. They are designed to detect individual patients' problems and as such are more readily interpreted in clinically meaningful ways. They also provide a basis for shared clinical decision-making between the patient and clinician, identifying patients' treatment priorities and facilitating the setting of realistic treatment goals. There may be opportunities to combine these approaches with short standardised measures that include "screening" questions. Further evaluation of the performance of individualised measures in clinical practice is required. This should be paralleled by developments in statistical methods to analyse individualised data.

Research

A number of questions about the clinical utility of quality of life measures remain unanswered. First, are our existing measures of quality of life appropriate and adequate for clinical practice or are new measures required? Answering this question will involve an evaluation of existing measures in clinical settings with appropriate psychometric assessment of their performance in individual patients over time. This raises the second question, which relates to the definition and assessment of change in quality of life in individual patients. How do existing measures take account of changes in expectations, adaptation, and normalisation when assessing change in quality of life? (See Chapter 2.) The third question is about the clinical interpretation of quality of life measures. What constitutes an important change in quality of life? And to whom is it important? Answering these questions will enable existing quality of life measures to be "calibrated" with respect to thresholds for intervention, thus helping to communicate to individual patients and their families better information about the likely individual benefits (or lack of benefits) from treatment.

> **Box 7.4 Future issues for research and education**
>
> - Studies that evaluate the introduction and utility of quality of life measures in routine practice are urgently needed.
> - Work is needed to better understand the clinical significance of changes in quality of life scores, so these can be better interpreted in the future.
> - Education of clinical staff should include training in the use and interpretation of quality of life measures as part of the routine assessment, just as staff are currently trained in history taking and laboratory tests.
> - Work is needed to further develop simple patient-centred measures, their analysis and interpretation and combination with simple screening quality of life components.

Acknowledgements

We thank our colleagues in the Interdisciplinary Research Group in Palliative and Person Centred Care at King's College London, in particular Peter Robinson, Barry Gibson, Stanley Gelbier, Robert Dunlop, Julia Addington-Hall, Lalit Kalra and Alan Turner-Smith, who have participated in discussions and commented on an earlier draft of this work. Alison Carr's post is funded by the Arthritis Research Campaign.

References

1. Bowling A. *Measuring disease. A review of quality of life measurement scales*. Milton Keynes: Open University, 1995.
2. Rosser RM. A history of the development of health indices. In: Smith GT, ed. *Measuring the social benefits of medicine*. London: Office of Health Economics, 1985.
3. Higginson I. Clinical teams, general practice, audit and outcomes. In: Delamothe T, ed. *Outcomes into clinical practice*. London: British Medical Association Books, 1994.
4. Stowers K, Hughes RA, Carr AJ. Information exchange between patients and health professionals: consultation styles of rheumatologists and nurse practitioners. *Arthritis Rheum* 1999;**42**(suppl):388.
5. Maguire P, Walsh S, Jeacock J, Kingston R. Physical and psychological needs of patients dying from colo-rectal cancer. *Palliative Med* 1999;**13**:45–50.

6. Maguire P, Booth K, Elliot C, Jones B. Helping health care professionals involved in cancer care acquire key interviewing skills: the impact of workshops. *Eur J Cancer* 1996;**32A**:1486–9.
7. Higginson I, McCarthy M. Measuring symptoms in terminal cancer: are pain dyspnoea controlled? *J Roy Soc Med* 1989;**82**: 264–7.
8. Higginson I. *Clinical audit in palliative care.* Oxford: Radcliffe Medical Press, 1993.
9. Mount BM and Scott JF. Whither hospice evaluation? *J Chronic Dis* 1983;**36**:731–6.
10. Feinstein AR. Benefits and obstacles for development of health status assessment measures in clinical settings. *Med Care* 1992; **30**(suppl):50.
11. Deyo RA, Carter WB. Strategies for improving and expanding the application of health status measures in clinical settings: a researcher-developer viewpoint. *Med Care* 1992;**30**(suppl):176.
12. Thornicroft G, Slade M. Are routine outcome measures feasible in mental health? *Qual Health Care* 2000;**9**:84.
13. Aaronson NK, Ahmedzai S, Bergman B *et al.* The European Organisation for Research and Treatment of Cancer QLQ-C30: a quality of life instrument for use in international clinical trials in oncology. *J Natl Cancer Inst* 1993;**85**(5):365–75.
14. Fitzpatrick R, Davey C, Buxton MJ, Jones DR. Evaluating patient-based outcome measures for use in clinical trials. *Health Technol Assess* 1998;**2**(14):1–74.
15. Carr AJ. A patient-centred approach to evaluation and treatment in rheumatoid arthritis: the development of a clinical tool to measure patient-perceived handicap. *Br J Rheumatol* 1996;**35**: 921–32.
16. Higginson I, McCarthy M. Validity of a measure of palliative care – comparison with a quality of life index. *Palliative Med* 1994;**8**(4):282–90.
17. Bruera E, Kuehn N, Miller M, Selmser P and MacMillan K. The Edmonton symptom assessment system (ESAS): a simple method for the assessment of palliative care patients. *J Palliative Care* 1991;**7**(2):6–9.
18. Hearn J, Higginson IJ. Validation of a core outcome measure for palliative care – The palliative care outcome scale (The POS). *Qual Health Care* 1999;**8**:219–27.
19. Patterson C. Measuring outcomes in primary care: a patient-centred outcome measure, MYMOP, compared with the SF-36 health survey. *BMJ* 1996;**312**:1016–20.
20. Instituto Nazionale Tumori Psycho-oncology Teams. *Global Directory for Psycho-oncology Programs.* www.qlmed.org/psico-oncologo.html

21. Davies HTO, Nutley SM, Mannion R. Organisational culture and quality of health care. *Qual Health Care* 2000;**9**:111–19.
22. Higginson IJ, Jefferys P, Hodgson C. Outcome measures for routine use in dementia services: some practical considerations. *Qual Health Care* 1997;**6**:120–24.
23. Carr AJ, Thompson PW, Young A. Do health status measures have a role in rheumatology: a survey of rheumatologists' use of and attitudes towards health status measures in the UK. *Arthritis Rheum* 1996;**39**:2615.
24. Kirwan JR, Chaput de Saintonge DM, Joyce CRB, Currey HLF. Clinical judgement in rheumatoid arthritis. II Judging "current disease activity" in rheumatoid arthritis. *Ann Rheum Dis* 1983;**42**:648–51.
25. Kazis LE, Callahan LF, Meenan RF, Pincus T. Health status reports in the care of patients with rheumatoid arthritis. *J Clin Epidemiol* 1990;**43**:1243–53.
26. Crombie IK, Davies HTO. Missing link in the audit cycle. *Qual Health Care* 1993;**2**:47–8.
27. Higginson IJ, Hearn J, Webb D. Audit in palliative care: does practice change? *Eur J Cancer Care* 1996;**5**:233–6.
28. O'Boyle CA, McGee H, Hickey A, O'Malley K, Joyce CRB. Individual quality of life in patients undergoing hip replacement. *Lancet* 1992;**339**:1088–91.
29. Ruta A, Garatt AM. The Patient Generated Index Quality of Life. *Med Care* 1994;**32**:1109–26.

8: Measuring the impact of assistive technologies on quality of life: can rehabilitation professionals rise to the challenge?

JANE K SEALE AND ALAN R TURNER-SMITH

Summary points

- Rehabilitation professionals have frequently claimed that assistive technologies enhance quality of life, but until recently there had been little agreement on how to define quality of life within the context of assistive technologies and how to measure the impact of assistive technologies on quality of life.
- Recent work on assistive technology-related quality of life has focused on three kinds of measurement tools: general health-related quality of life instruments, participation-oriented instruments, and specially designed assistive technology instruments.
- Generic health-related quality of life instruments have produced mixed results about the impact of assistive technologies and the applicability of the instruments to the field of assistive technology has not always been adequately addressed.
- Although the use of participation-oriented instruments is attractive to rehabilitation professionals, there is at the moment little data on the use of such tools within the field of assistive technology.
- Some rehabilitation professionals are developing and testing specific assistive technology-related tools. Their attraction lies in their validity and reliability being tested with a range of assistive technology users.
- Future research and debate should consider whether rehabilitation professionals should use specific tools or just a battery of tools that includes more general quality of life assessments.

Introduction

Assistive technology is an umbrella term for any device or system that allows an individual to perform a task they would otherwise be unable to do or increases the ease and safety with which the task can be performed. Assistive technologies include wheelchairs, communication aids, computers, and aids to daily living such as reachers. This chapter uses the example of assistive technology as a case study that reflects the conceptual and methodological evolution of quality of life research in other areas of medicine.

In the 1980s and 1990s advocates of assistive technology frequently claimed that it could improve patient quality of life. But what they actually meant by quality of life varied considerably. Claims surrounding quality of life were frequently linked to notions of increased independence, productivity or social participation. For example, in 1984 Kornblugh talked about the role assistive technologies could play for older people and predicted that they:

> will want more than a decent place to live and enough to eat; they will want more independence, continued productivity and be less tolerant of custodial care. In other words, they will want an enhanced quality of life in their twilight years.[1]

While outlining the importance of developing more and better assistive technologies in order to improve the quality of life for disabled and elderly people, Cooper argued:

> with the development and appropriate application of proper assistive technology, persons with disabilities can lead more active and productive lives. The ultimate goal is to develop and appropriately apply proper assistive technologies to ameliorate problems faced by persons with disabilities and to allow them to participate fully in every aspect of society.[2]

Around the mid 1990s rehabilitation professionals began to acknowledge that they needed to consider outcomes that would adequately and appropriately measure the impact of assistive technologies on quality of life. This acknowledgement was linked to concerns about why some patients abandoned assistive technologies. It was important to explore why individuals decided to accept or reject different types of assistive technologies and this work was critical to improving the effectiveness of assistive technology interventions and enhancing individuals' quality of life.[3]

In attempting to explore the impact of assistive technologies on quality of life, rehabilitation professionals have used a number of instruments from general health-related quality of life instruments, participation-oriented instruments to specially designed assistive technology-specific measures. We will consider these three approaches in turn.

Using general health-related quality of life instruments

Some practitioners have attempted to explore the impact of assistive technologies on their patients' quality of life by using pre-existing generic health-related quality of life instruments. Reported instruments include the SQUALA, Rand SF-36 and EuroQol.

The SQUALA (Subjective Quality of Life Assessment) was used to assess the influence of barrier-free houses on the quality of life of 34 physically disabled people living in the Czech Republic.[4] The SQUALA requires respondents to evaluate the importance of 23 domains including health, physical independence, love, work, and money.[5] Despite arguing for improvements in the measurement of quality of life they did not consider the generalisability of the SQUALA, which appears to have been developed for use in psychiatric settings.

The Rand SF-36 was one of four outcome measures used to study the impact of wheelchairs on 24 older people.[6] The Rand SF-36 is a self-administered generic health assessment tool consisting of 36 items. Eight health concepts are measured, including physical function, role limitation due to physical or mental health, bodily pain, social health, and mental health. Rand SF-36 showed that the wheelchairs increased quality of life in the areas of role and social functioning. In another study, the Rand SF-36 did not associate hip replacements with improved quality of life.[7] Participants with no hip replacement reported higher scores on the SF-36 for physical function.

Adaptation of generic measures

Some rehabilitation professionals are unhappy with the medical orientation of generic instruments such as the Rand SF-36 and EuroQol.

EuroQol-5D measures health-related quality of life in five dimensions: mobility, self-care, usual activities, pain/discomfort, and anxiety/depression.[8] One group has adapted EuroQol by adding two dimensions. The Efficiency of Assistive Technology and Services (EATS-2D) enquires about social participation and mobility (as distinct from locomotion).[9] The same group has also developed the EATS-VAS, a thermometer-type scale to rate the impact of functional disabilities on perceived restrictions in performing everyday activities. Although the EATS group has not considered changes to the validity and reliability that might arise from adapting the EuroQol, their tools have been used in conjunction with the EuroQol in a number of studies. For example, GelderBlom and colleagues included the EuroQol and EATS-VAS in a battery of assessments to evaluate the impact of the MANUS robot arm on 35 disabled Dutch users.[10] Quality of life was higher for long-term MANUS users compared to non-users. For 10 new users of MANUS, no significant difference was found in the reported quality of life prior to and after the arrival of the robot arm.

In an attempt to develop a socio-economic model for assessing telephone and videophone relay services, Gotherstrom and Persson administered a number of tools, including the EuroQol-5D and EATS-2D, to four people who had been deaf since birth.[11] Hellbom and Persson included the EuroQol-5D and EATS-VAS in a study designed to compare the performance of two assessors.[12] They asked two assessors to assess clients with mobility problems who had been prescribed assistive technology solutions. One assessor had prescribed the assistive technology device; the other was an independent assessor. The "prescriber" ascribed stronger effects to the assistive technology solutions, suggesting that independent assessors should evaluate the effectiveness of assistive technologies.

Measures focussing on handicap and participation

In urging rehabilitation professionals to examine the potential of health-related quality of life instruments carefully, Oldridge considered medically orientated instruments as not wholly adequate for outcome measurement in assistive technology.[13] More targeted instruments may need to be developed. Some rehabilitation professionals see social participation as a key dimension for more specific measurement. For example, Kemp administered four measures, including a 16-item community activities checklist, to 110 ageing persons with disability.[14] He argued for greater attention to be paid to the impacts of community activities that gave pleasure, success, and meaning to the individual's life. Similarly, the EATS group were dissatisfied with the EuroQol instrument because it did not adequately measure social participation and their EATS-2D amendment was a step toward a more targeted instrument.

The LIFE-H instrument attempts to assess the quality of social participation by using life habit as an operational construct of social participation.[15] Life habit was defined as a daily activity or social role valued by the person and his/her socio-cultural context. The instrument has short and long forms with 69 and 240 items respectively. Both cover 12 categories of life habits, six of which refer to activities of daily living and six to social roles. People respond to each item on the scale by marking the degree of difficulty and the types of required assistance (technical aid or human assistance). In describing its application to the field of assistive technology, Noreau and colleagues argue that when people are unable to accomplish their life habits their social participation is restricted (they are handicapped).[16] Noreau and colleagues suggest that the LIFE-H is a potential tool to determine the impact of assistive technology provision on social participation. Despite this suggestion, the LIFE-H has not yet been extensively tested in the assistive technology field. Nevertheless, the tool could be attractive to rehabilitation professionals for three main reasons. First, it has been tested with a wide range of populations including spinal cord injury, traumatic brain injury, cerebral palsy, and myotonic dystrophy. Second, it is not a profession-specific tool. Third, and perhaps most important, the theory underpinning the tool is deeply rooted in the accepted international understanding of disability and handicap (as defined by the World Health Organization's Classification System: ICDH-2, now ICF) where social participation is seen as the result of an interaction between an individual's characteristics and his/her environment.

Assistive technology-specific instruments

Whilst the LIFE-H tool has potential, it was not developed specifically for the field of assistive technology. One tool that has been developed specifically for this field is the PIADS (Psychosocial Impact of Assistive Devices Scale).[17] The development of this tool has been underpinned by the assertion that an assistive device will promote good quality of life for the user to the extent to which it makes the user feel competent, confident, and inclined to exploit life's possibilities.

The PIADS is a 26-item self-rating questionnaire designed to measure user perceptions of how assistive devices affect quality of life. It is intended to be a user-centred measure applicable to virtually all forms of assistive technology. The PIADS describes user perceptions along three dimensions: adaptability, competence and self-esteem. Adaptability refers to the enabling and liberating effects of the device. Example items are eagerness to try new things and ability to adapt to the activities of daily living. Competence refers to the impact of the device on functional independence, performance, and productivity. Example items are efficiency, independence, and usefulness. Self-esteem refers to the extent to which the device has affected emotional wellbeing. Example items for this dimension are frustration and happiness.

The adaptability dimension reflects notions of social participation while the competence dimension reflects notions of productivity and independence. All these concepts are significant and relevant outcomes of assistive technology. The validity and reliability of PIADS was originally established with eyeglass and contact lens wearers. Preliminary studies have also been conducted with wheelchair users.

Early evaluations suggest that PIADS has the potential to be a useful user-centred indicator of quality of life in assistive technology. The inclusion of self-esteem as a dimension within the PIADS tool is novel given that the impact of assistive technologies on self-esteem is not widely discussed. Sherer found that using a personal computer affected self-esteem among nursing home residents in Israel, but the effect was small compared to that on morale and life satisfaction.[18]

PIADS is also being used to explore questions applicable to the wider quality of life research community such as the influence of patient expectations and the use of proxies. PIADS was used to compare the perceived psychosocial impact of electronic assistive devices on a group of device users with the anticipated impact of electronic assistive devices on a group who had not yet received these devices.[19] Anticipated impacts were similar to those experienced, which indicates realistic expectations about the devices. User and caregiver assessments of the psychosocial impact of assistive devices have also been compared with PIADS.[20] Correlations between the groups suggest that caregivers' assessments of psychosocial benefits could be used as proxies to evaluate assistive technology.

Conclusion

In order to explore the impact of assistive technologies on quality of life, rehabilitation professionals have used, adapted, and designed a variety of quality of life instruments. Generic health-related quality of life instruments have produced mixed results about the impact of assistive technologies. Furthermore, the applicability of the instruments has not always been adequately addressed. Some rehabilitation professionals have called for specific or focused quality of life instruments, in particular those that focus on social participation. There is little data on the use of tools such as LIFE-H in assistive technology. Finally, some rehabilitation professionals are developing and testing specific assistive technology-related tools such as the PIADS. Their attraction lies in their validity and reliability being tested with a range of assistive technology users. Research and debate should consider whether rehabilitation professionals should use only specific tools such as PIADS or a battery of tools that include more general quality of life assessments.

References

1. Kornbluh M. Computer and telecommunications applications to enhance the quality of life of our elderly citizens. In: Robinson PK, Livingston J, Birren JE, eds. *Aging and Technological Advances*. New York: Plenum Press, 1984, pp. 425–31.
2. Cooper RA. Forging a new future: a call for integrating people with disabilities into rehabilitation engineering. *Technol Disability* 1995;4:81–5.
3. Scherer M. Outcomes of assistive technology use on quality of life. *Disability Rehabil* 1996;18:439–48.
4. Votava J, Brabcova L, Hornikova J. Assistive device's application and its influence on quality of life in people with severe disability, living in barrier-free houses in the Czech Republic. In: Marincek C, Buhler C, Knops H, Andrich R, eds. *Assistive Technology – Added Value to the Quality of Life*. Amsterdam: IOS Press, 2001, pp. 639–50.
5. Zanotti M, Pringeuy D. A method for quality of life assessment in psychiatry: the SQUALA (Subjective Quality of Life Analysis). *Qual Life Newsletter* 1992;4:6.
6. Bursick TM, Trefler E, Fitzgerald S, Joseph R. Wheelchair seating and positioning outcomes in the elderly nursing home population. In: Winters J, ed. *Technology for the New Millennium*. Proceedings of the RESNA 2000 Annual Conference. Arlington, VA: RESNA Press, 2000, pp. 316–18.
7. Frost KL, Fitzgerald SG, Bertocci GE, Mumin MC. Functional status and well-being following total hip replacement rehabilitation as measured using the SF-36. In: Winters J, ed. *Technology for the New Millennium*. Proceedings of the RESNA 2000 Annual Conference. Arlington, VA: RESNA Press, 2000, pp. 325–7.

8. EuroQol Business Management Group. *EuroQol-5D User Guide*. Rotterdam, 1996.

9. Persson J, Andrich R, Beekum T *et al*. EuroQOL, EATS-2D and EATS-VAS: quality of life of disabled persons. In: Marincek C, Buhler C, Knops H, Andrich R, eds. *Assistive Technology – Added Value to the Quality of Life*. Amsterdam: IOS Press, 2001, pp. 606–7.

10. GelderBlom GJ, De Witte L, Van Soest R *et al*. Evaluation of the MANUS robot manipulator. In: Marincek C, Buhler C, Knops H, Andrich R, eds. *Assistive Technology – Added Value to the Quality of Life*. Amsterdam: IOS Press, 2001, pp. 268–73.

11. Gotherstrom U-C, Persson J. Text telephone relay service and video phone relay service – quantification of benefits for the user. In: Marincek C, Buhler C, Knops H, Andrich R, eds. *Assistive Technology – Added Value to the Quality of Life*. Amsterdam: IOS Press, 2001, pp. 575–9.

12. Hellbom G, Persson J. Estimating user benefits of assistive technology and services – on the importance of independent assessors. In: Marincek C, Buhler C, Knops H, Andrich R, eds. *Assistive Technology – Added Value to the Quality of Life*. Amsterdam: IOS Press, 2001, pp. 551–4.

13. Oldridge NB. Outcomes measurement: health-related quality of life. *Assist Technol* 1996;**8**:82–93.

14. Kemp BJ. Quality of life while aging with a disability. *Assist Technol* 1999;**11**:158–63.

15. Fougeyrollas P, Noreau L, Bergeron H *et al*. Social consequences of long-term impairments and disabilities: conceptual approach and assessment of handicap. *Int J Rehabil Res* 1998;**21**:127–41.

16. Noreau L, Fougeyrollas P, Vincent C. The LIFE-H: assessment of the quality of social participation. In: Marincek C, Buhler C, Knops H, Andrich R, eds. *Assistive Technology – Added Value to the Quality of Life*. Amsterdam: IOS Press, 2001, pp. 604–5.

17. Jutai J. Quality of life impact of assistive technology. *Rehabil Eng* 1999;**14**:2–7.

18. Sherer M. The impact of using personal computers on the lives of nursing home residents. *Phys Occup Ther Geriatr* 1996;**14**:13–31.

19. Jutai J, Rigby P, Ryan S, Stickel S. Psychosocial impact of electronic aids to daily living. *Assist Technol* 2000;**12**:123–31.

20. Jutai J, Woolrich W, Campbell K. User care-giver agreement on perceived psychosocial impact of assistive devices. In: Winters J, ed. *Technology for the New Millennium*. Proceedings of the RESNA 2000 Annual Conference. Arlington, VA: RESNA Press, 2000, pp. 328–30.

9: How to choose a quality of life measure

PETER G ROBINSON, ALISON J CARR
AND IRENE J HIGGINSON

Summary points

- Selecting an appropriate quality of life measure from the many available can be a complex process.
- The choice of measure is determined by:
  - why you want to measure quality of life
  - whose quality of life you want to measure
  - what questions you want it to answer.
- Generic measures assess quality of life across different populations or with different diseases. Their broad applicability means that they may ignore domains important to specific groups.
- Specific measures focus on problems associated with specific situations and are more likely to discriminate between specific groups and respond to change.
- Some specific issues need to be considered:
  - Does the measure contain items relevant to your purpose and participants? Will it be able to measure across the range of disease severity that you are interested in? Measures developed in other countries require both linguistic and contextual translation. Can the scores you obtain be analysed to answer your question?

Introduction

The measurement of health-related quality of life is concerned with quantifying the judgements people make to describe their experiences of health and illness. This emphasis on the subjective experience of the impact of disease on everyday life derives from two related factors. First, our growing knowledge of the relevance of the social determinants and consequences of health and disease means that we must find ways of measuring health in subjective, personal, and social terms.

Second, we recognise that healthcare not only aims to save life, but also to prevent and reduce these consequences of disease.

Numerous authors have listed potential applications of this type of information.[1-7] The ideas expressed by these authors are broadly compatible and can be summarised in the framework of political, theoretical, and practical applications outlined by Locker (Table 9.1).[3]

New quality of life measures are constantly added to the numerous assortment that already exists and selecting the most appropriate measure for a specific research or clinical situation can be a difficult and time consuming process. Chapter 7 of this book considered the use of quality of life measures in clinical practice. Choice of a quality of life measure was discussed in clinical settings focussing on practicability and psychometric properties such as validity and reliability. These aspects of an instrument are essential in any setting, but the qualities required of an instrument will also vary depending on the purpose for which it is being used.[8] For example, measures used in a population-based survey must be concise, efficient, and broadly applicable, whereas a measure used to detect the benefit of treatments for a particular disease will need to detect the very specific social and functional consequences of this condition and respond to the changes brought about by treatment. It follows that a measure designed for one purpose may not be useful for the other.

This chapter will discuss those factors that should be considered when choosing which quality of life measure to use for specific situations. In this discussion, emphasis is placed on the purpose of measurement and how that influences the suitability and appropriateness of different quality of life measures. The essential psychometric properties of quality of life measures have been described in some detail in Chapter 7 and will only be mentioned here in the context of how the purpose of measurement might affect them.

Why are you measuring quality of life?

There are three major considerations when determining the purpose of measurement.

Table 9.1 Applications of health-related quality of life measures

Political		Seeking resources and influencing policy makers
		Harnessing public opinion
		Encouraging lay involvement in policy making
Theoretical		Identifying factors that influence health
		Exploring models of health
		Elucidating the relationships between different aspects of health
Practical	Research	Use as outcome when assessing the effectiveness and efficiency of healthcare
	Public Health	Describing and monitoring illness in populations
		Planning, monitoring, and evaluating services
		Needs assessment and prioritising
		Encouraging greater lay participation in healthcare
	Clinical Practice	Facilitating communication among healthcare workers and patients
		Assisting patients towards autonomy
		Screening for, identifying, and prioritising patient problems
		Identifying patient preferences
		Monitoring and evaluating individual patient care
		Identifying which patients have the propensity to benefit from treatment
		Clinical audit
		Marketing services

- What are you using the quality of life measure for?
- Whose quality of life are you measuring?
- What question are you asking (i.e. how will the data be analysed)?

What are you using the quality of life measure for?

Quality of life measures can be used for a wide range of purposes: to quantify the quality of life of populations; to assess the relative impact of different diseases; to evaluate the effectiveness of treatment in clinical trials; to measure the quality of care; and to identify specific problems in individual patients in clinical practice and measure the effectiveness of treatment in addressing those problems. Given the range of uses, it seems unlikely that any one quality of life measure will be equally appropriate or accurate in all situations. The purpose of measurement places specific requirements on the content, structure, and psychometric properties of quality of life measures.

Generic versus specific measures

Quality of life measures can be categorised as generic or condition/disease-specific.[8] Generic measures are designed to assess general health-related quality of life across different populations or with different diseases. Their content is necessarily broad and covers those aspects of quality of life that are most important to most people, such as physical and social function and freedom from pain. The broad applicability of generic measures allows comparisons between groups or people with different conditions, such as in studies of populations or comparative studies of the relative impact of different diseases. Many generic measures have been developed and their psychometric properties have been comprehensively evaluated.[9] Examples of generic quality of life measures include the Nottingham Health Profile, SF-36, EuroQoL, and the World Health Organization Quality of Life measure. The broad applicability of generic measures means that they may ignore some domains that are important to specific groups of people such as those in a given age range or with a specific disease. By omitting these domains, the instruments may lack the precision to discriminate between specific groups of people or be responsive to changes brought about by treatment. This may limit their usefulness in some clinical settings or clinical trials.

Disease-specific measures address these problems by focussing on particular problems associated with specific anatomical divisions, body systems or diseases.[10] Their focus on impacts of a particular condition means that they are more likely to discriminate between specific groups and respond to change. They will also rule out unnecessary and irrelevant items. As a result, they may be more responsive to change within patient groups and, therefore, more suitable for use in clinical trials or with individual patients in clinical practice. Examples of disease-specific measures include the rheumatoid arthritis quality of life scale and the European Organization for Research and Treatment of Cancer QLQ-C30.[11,12] The specific focus of these measures on one group of patients precludes their use in cross-disease comparisons or population studies and might mean that other important consequences of disease are not detected.[8]

The debate about the relative advantages and disadvantages of generic and specific measures persists. In some situations valid and reliable generic measures perform as well as specific ones,[13] but there are situations where the added precision of a specific measure renders it more sensitive to differences.[14] One solution is to use a combination of generic and specific measures that confers the advantages of both.[15,16] Some measures, for example the European Organization for Research and Treatment of Cancer Quality of Life questionnaire, have a core set of items and add-on system-specific modules.[17] The SF-36 also has an increasing number of disease-specific add-on items. Alternatively, generic and disease-specific measures may be used in tandem.[18,19] The Sickness Impact Profile and the SF-36 are often used in this way.[20,21] Whilst sensitive and comprehensive assessment is ideal, it can only be achieved using longer and more demanding instruments. In turn, greater complexity will result in lower completion rates and more errors. A suitable compromise must be reached between adequacy of data and researcher and participant burden.

The content of the measure

The content of the measure will also determine its usefulness in different settings. Content validity is concerned with whether the domains and level of questions are appropriate for the setting and participants being studied. For example, an item that asked whether one could move without assistance would not be suitable for assessing the fitness of sportsmen. Although the domain of interest is mobility, the level of questions one would ask a patient with severe osteoarthritis is very different from that required for a sportsman. Very particularly, the items of the instruments must be likely to be responsive to the consequences of the condition or treatment in the people under study.

Quality of life instruments are developed by selecting a number of items from a larger panel of potential items. There are two methods for selecting those items to be included in the final measure. The first is based on psychometric theory and uses statistical methods (often factor analysis) to mathematically reduce the number of items to be included in a questionnaire to a manageable number that does not include statistically redundant or overlapping items.[22] Whilst this is the traditional approach, it can result in measures from which items that are important to patients are excluded, thereby reducing its validity and responsiveness. For example, this approach to the development of the Nottingham Health Profile resulted in the removal of items of interest to patients, particularly those relating to less severe but commonly experienced impacts. This mathematical control of item selection produced a very insensitive measure: in general populations the majority of people scored zero.[23]

The second approach (the item impact method) selects items, not on the basis of their statistical relationship to one another, but on the basis of their importance to patients. Juniper and colleagues developed a disease-specific quality of life instrument for people with asthma by administering a large pool of items to a patient sample.[22] The items used in the final instrument were those relating to problems whose impact on the patients was frequent and severe. This method produced a measure with rather different items from those featured in one developed using factor analysis. More recently both the item-impact and factor analysis methods have been used in combination.[24]

This approach had been adopted recently in evaluations of oral health-related quality of life. Short forms of the Oral Health Impact Profile were derived from the original panel of

49 items using the item impact method in both Canada and the United Kingdom.[25,26] The new short forms were compared with each other and to an existing short form derived using regression analysis.[27] The British and Canadian short forms were similar but differed substantially from the existing version. Furthermore, both new short forms had better cross-sectional psychometric properties and the British version was more responsive than the original version.[28]

Whose quality of life are you measuring?

Whose quality of life you want to measure will naturally determine the choice of instrument. Ease of completion, questionnaire length, complexity of the scoring, and whether it is interviewer-administered or self-completed will determine which measures are most appropriate for clinical practice, which can be used in postal surveys, and which can be accommodated in a clinical trial. In addition, the complexity of some instruments precludes their use with people who are infirm or who have limited cognitive ability. For people who are visually impaired or illiterate, traditional paper and pencil, self-completed measures are not appropriate and alternative modes of administration (interviewer-administered, interactive computerised measures, and so on) are needed.

When considering whose quality of life you want to measure, it is also important to be aware of the provenance of the different quality of life measures, i.e. what population of patients/normal subjects was it developed in (age, gender, disease severity) and in what cultural context (has it been translated from a different language)?

Scaling of quality of life measures

Any measure is generally developed and tested within a particular population of patients or subjects. This means that the results of the psychometric testing (the validity, reliability, and responsiveness to change) will really only apply to that particular group and setting. Despite this, many "validated" measures are adopted for use in a variety of settings, some of which bear little relation to the original sample. This raises potential problems relating to the measure's ability to represent quality of life accurately in particular patients, groups or settings, and in its responsiveness to change in those settings. For example, a quality of life measure may have been developed in a group of patients with very severe disease with the result that the measure will only be able to quantify quality of life in patients with severe disease, no part of the scale representing patients with moderate or mild disease. Similarly, a measure developed only in patients with moderate disease may not include a range of items or scales of severity to capture the quality of life in patients with mild or severe disease. Measures that do not cover the whole range of disease severity in their items and scaling will be less responsive to change because of floor and ceiling effects (i.e. the scale will not identify improvement in patients with mild disease or deterioration in patients with severe disease). When selecting a quality of life measure, it is important to ensure that the population you propose to use the measure in is similar to the population who were involved in the development and validation of the measure. If there is a significant difference, you may have to do some validation work in your own population to ensure that the measure retains its validity, reliability, and responsiveness.

Cross-cultural use of quality of life measures

Most of the available quality of life measures have been originally developed in one cultural setting and then translated for use in other contexts. Where this process involves rigorous translation and back-translation of the questions it ensures the semantic equivalence of the measures but, unless there is some assessment of the conceptual equivalence, the validity of the measure may be compromised. In other words, semantic equivalence means that the items on the questionnaire say the same things in different languages but it may be that they do not adequately capture quality of life in that new cultural setting.[29] One measure that has overcome these problems, enabling quality of life to be measured and compared across many cultural settings is the WHOQOL.[30] This measure was simultaneously developed in several countries so that the different versions all measure quality of life within the same general domains (daily activities, spirituality, emotional wellbeing, and so on) but the specific items used to capture quality of life in those domains differs depending on the cultural setting.

Individualised measures

Individualised quality of life measures (such as the Schedule for Evaluation of Individualised Quality of Life (SEIQOL) and the Patient Generated Index (PGI)) allow patients to specify those aspects of quality of life of most importance to them and to rate the impact of their condition on those aspects.[31,32] They have been developed as a consequence of the argument that quality of life is necessarily specific to individuals and cannot be adequately represented by standardised measures that impose a general definition of quality of life. Chapter 3 considers the relative merits of individualised and standardised quality of life measures. They may be more appropriate than standardised measures in clinical practice where the aim is to identify the specific quality of life issues of individual patients. Problems with aggregating the scores to enable between group comparisons have so far limited their use in research.

What question are you asking?

In analytical terms, quality of life measures may be used for three purposes.[33] Discriminative measures are used to distinguish between individuals or groups, typically in cross-sectional studies to quantify or compare the burden of illness. Evaluative measures assess change over time, for example in a randomised controlled trial. Finally, predictive measures are used to classify individuals into categories pre-defined by existing criteria; for example, when screening for disease.

The psychometric properties required of an instrument will vary according to its purpose.[33] Furthermore, validity for one purpose does not imply adequate validity for others. Discriminative measures require good cross-sectional construct validity and test-retest reliability. These features ensure that there will be large differences between different population groups, which are stable over time. Good criterion validity is, by definition, essential in a predictive index, as is test-retest reliability. Several authors recommend that a test used in day to day practice as a decision making tool should have very high internal consistency (reliability), with a Cronbach's alpha coefficient greater than 0.90, although if the measure provides a profile of quality of life in several separate and different domains, high internal consistency is not an appropriate test.[19] In an evaluative instrument the cross-sectional construct validity is less important than the test-retest reliability and responsiveness (see Chapter 10 on data analysis).

Because quality of life is multidimensional, instruments that collect data on several domains may present the data for each domain separately or may summarise the data as a small number of summary statistics. There are profound interpre-tational and analytical consequences of each approach, which are discussed in Chapter 10. To some extent, these consequences can be anticipated. For example, in anticipating the course of a disease or treatment, is an impact in one domain likely to be replaced with another? If so, then a measure that uses a simple summary statistic is likely to mask this change.

One other aspect of an instrument often overlooked is the time frame. Items in questionnaires or instruments often enquire about the impact of a disease over a given reference period. Again, the reference period must match the purpose of the study. In a condition that varies over time, a longer reference period is more likely to provide more reliable data. Yet a long reference period will be unsuitable for short-term evaluations. For example, the reference periods for data collected at baseline and follow up in a trial should not overlap. Similarly, a long reference period may not be sufficiently precise to detect acute impacts of disease.[34]

Discussion and future directions

Choosing a quality of life measure for use in clinical practice or research is fraught with potential difficulties. The process could be significantly simplified if the developers of scales produced guides for their use that specified in which setting the questionnaire could be used, with which groups of patients there was evidence for its validity and reliability, and what sort of analysis it could be subjected to.

References

1. Ware JE Jr, Brook RH, Davies AR, Lohr KN. Choosing measures of health status for individuals in general populations. *Am J Public Health* 1981;**71**:620–25.
2. Sheiham A, Maizels JE, Cushing AM. The concept of need in dental care. *Int Dent J* 1982;**32**:265–8.
3. Locker D. Applications of self-reported assessments of oral health outcomes. *J Dent Educ* 1996;**60**:494–500.
4. Weintraub JA. Uses of oral health related quality of life measures in Public Health. *Community Dent Health* 1998;**15**:8–12.
5. Corson MA, Boyd T, Kind P, Allen PF, Steele JG. Measuring oral health: does your treatment really make a difference? *Br Dent J* 1999;**187**:481–4.
6. McGrath C, Bedi R. The value and use of "quality of life" measures in the primary dental care setting. *Primary Dent Care* 1999;**6**:53–7.
7. Hayry M. Measuring the quality of life: Why, how what. In: Joyce CRB, O'Boyle CA, McGee H, eds. *Individual quality of life. Approaches to conceptualisation and assessment.* Amsterdam: Harwood Academic Press, 1999, pp. 9–27.
8. Patrick DL, Deyo RA. Generic and disease-specific measures in assessing health status and quality of life. *Med Care* 1989;**27**: 217–32.
9. Bowling A. *Measuring health. A review of quality of life measurement scales*, 2nd ed. Buckingham. Open University Press, 1997.
10. Bowling A. *Measuring disease. A review of disease-specific quality of life measurement scales*. Buckingham: Open University Press, 1995.
11. Aaronson NK, Ahmedzai S, Bergman B *et al*. The European Organization for Research and Treatment of Cancer QLQ-C30: a quality-of-life instrument for use in international clinical trials in oncology. *J Natl Cancer Inst* 1993;**85**:365–76.
12. de Jong Z, van der Heijde D, McKenna SP, Whalley D. The reliability and construct validity of the RAQoL: a rheumatoid arthritis-specific quality of life instrument. *Br J Rheumatol* 1997;**36**:878–83.
13. Parkerson GR, Jr, Connis RT, Broadhead WE *et al*. Disease-specific versus generic measurement of health-related quality of

life in insulin-dependent diabetic patients. *Med Care* 1993;**31**: 629–39.

14. Allen PF, McMillan AS, Walshaw D, Locker D. A comparison of the validity of generic- and disease-specific measures in the assessment of oral health-related quality of life. *Community Dent Oral Epidemiol* 1999;**27**:344–52.

15. Osoba D. Measuring the effect of cancer on health-related quality of life. *Pharmacoecon* 1995;**7**:308–19.

16. Scott DL, Garrood T. Quality of life measures: use and abuse. *Baillieres Best Pract Res Clin Rheumatol* 2000;**14**:663–87.

17. Fayers P, Bottomley A. Quality of life research within the EORTC – the EORTC QLQ-C30. *Eur J Cancer* 2002;**38**(suppl 4):125–33.

18. Berzon RA. Understanding and using health-related quality of life instruments within clinical research studies. In: Staquet MJ, Hays RD, Fayers PM, eds. *Quality of life assessment in clinical trials. Methods and Practice.* Oxford: Oxford University Press, 1998, pp. 3–15.

19. Osoba D. Guidelines for measuring health-related quality of life in clinical trials. In: Staquet MJ, Hays RD, Fayers PM, eds. *Quality of life assessment in clinical trials.* Oxford: Oxford University Press, 1998, pp. 19–35.

20. Dougherty DD, Baer L, Cosgrove GR *et al.* Prospective long-term follow-up of 44 patients who received cingulotomy for treatment-refractory obsessive-compulsive disorder. *Am J Psychiatry* 2002;**159**:269–75.

21. Bacon CG, Giovannucci E, Testa M, Glass TA, Kawachi I. The association of treatment-related symptoms with quality-of-life outcomes for localized prostate carcinoma patients. *Cancer* 2002;**94**:862–71.

22. Juniper EF, Guyatt GH, Streiner DL, King DR. Clinical impact versus factor analysis for quality of life questionnaire construction. *J Clin Epidemiol* 1997;**50**:233–8.

23. Hunt SM. The researcher's tale: a story of virtue lost and regained. In: Joyce CRB, O'Boyle CA, McGee H, eds. *Individual quality of life. Approaches to conceptualisation and assessment.* Amsterdam: Harwood Academic Press, 1999, pp. 225–32.

24. Cronin L, Guyatt G, Griffith L *et al.* Development of a health-related quality-of-life questionnaire (PCOSQ) for women with polycystic ovary syndrome (PCOS). *J Clin Endocrinol Metab* 1998;**83**:1976–87.

25. Slade GD, Spencer AJ. Development and evaluation of the Oral Health Impact Profile. *Community Dent Health* 1994;**11**:3–11.

26. Locker D, Allen FP. Developing short-form measures of oral health-related quality of life using the item-impact method. *J Dent Res* 2001;**80**:1146(abstr).

27. Slade GD. Derivation and validation of a short-form oral health impact profile. *Community Dent Oral Epidemiol* 1997;**25**:284–90.

28. Allen FP, Locker D. Measurement properties of a modified shortened version of the Oral Health Impact Profile. *J Dent Res* 2001;**80**:1146(abstr).

29. Deyo RA. Pitfalls in measuring the health status of Mexican Americans: comparative validity of the English and Spanish Sickness Impact Profile. *Am J Public Health* 1984;**74**:569–73.

30. Skevington S. Measuring quality of life in Britain. Introducing the WHOQOL-100. *J Psychosom Res* 1999;**47**:449–59.

31. O'Boyle CA, McGee H, Hickey A *et al. The schedule for the evaluation of individual quality of life. User manual.* Dublin: Royal College of Surgeons in Ireland, 1993.

32. Ruta D, Garratt A, Leng M, Russell I, MacDonald L. A new approach to the measurement of quality of life. The Patient-Generated Index. *Med Care* 1994;**32**:1109–26.

33. Worthington HV. Statistical aspects of measuring change in oral health status of older adults. *Community Dent Oral Epidemiol* 1998;**26**:48–51.

34. Robinson PG, Gibson B, Khan FA, Birnbaum W. Validity of two Oral Health Related Quality of Life measures in a UK setting. *Community Dent Oral Epidemiol* (in press).

10: Longitudinal analysis of quality of life data

PETER G ROBINSON AND NORA DONALDSON

Summary points

- Longitudinal analysis poses particular challenges for quality of life research.
- Participants may be lost, may remember events in a different light and can be conditioned by repeatedly completing questionnaires.
- Because the scores from a quality of life measure have no inherent meaning it may be necessary to define the minimum amount of change in quality of life that is important.
- Measures that summarise quality of life in a single value may mask important changes.
- An individual's internal scales of measuring quality of life may change (response shift).
- Response shift complicates analysis by making it difficult to distinguish between changes brought about by treatment or the progression of disease and other types of change.
- An understanding of response shift also provides new insights into longitudinal analysis.

Introduction

Longitudinal research involves data collection at several points in time and poses particular challenges for quality of life research.[1] Participants may be lost, may remember events in a different light (sample attrition and recall bias, respectively), and can be conditioned by repeatedly completing questionnaires. We also need to allow for the relative scope for improvement or deterioration among patients who may start off with different levels of quality of life. In addition, the principle of repeating measurements assumes that the measurement scale stays constant. "Response shift" hypothesises that an individual's internal scales of measurement change (see Chapter 2).[2,3]

This chapter discusses the analysis of longitudinal quality of life data. We focus principally on randomised controlled trials (RCTs) involving health-related quality of life data but also consider more generic studies. We also devote some attention to aspects of methodology and analysis.

Many of the difficulties that arise from general methodological errors are accentuated in quality of life research. Methodological challenges of a general nature are considered in many excellent texts and are beyond the scope of this chapter.

General aspects

Principles of longitudinal analysis in randomised controlled trialls

The simplest analytical approach involves data collection only twice – once before and once after treatment. This approach has intuitive appeal and the data are easier to interpret than comparisons at many time periods. However, before and after designs will oversimplify the analysis if the change in quality of life is transient or if it does not happen until after the follow up. Alternatively, treatments may have transitional negative effects that are slowly outweighed by the benefits of treatment. For these reasons the choice of endpoint is crucial.

The analytical approach typical of randomised controlled trials is to compare the outcome variables between the study and control groups. We would expect patients who start a trial with different levels of quality of life to respond differently. People with very good quality of life will have little scope for improvement and patients with extremely high or low scores will appear to moderate over time by regression to the mean. Furthermore, by accounting for the baseline value we increase the precision of the measures of treatment effects. For these reasons the outcomes are usually compared in relation to their baseline value.

Two methods can be used to account for the situation at baseline: to calculate the change as the difference between the baseline and follow-up values (unconditional analysis) or to adjust for the baseline score using analysis of covariance (conditional analysis).

Unconditional analysis of change scores presents several difficulties. Change scores acquire measurement errors at both baseline and follow up and do not account for regression to the mean. The effects of these errors are cumulative and may mask treatment effects unless the instrument is very reliable.[4] Conditional analysis is preferred because it adjusts for baseline values as a covariate.[5-7] The analysis of covariance assesses the association between the baseline and follow-up values and makes appropriate adjustment. This method also lends the opportunity to adjust for other variables that may be related to the outcome (confounders) as in a regression model. A word of caution is needed; there is a tendency to "overmodel" data and there should be a scientific case for each covariate employed.[8]

Values from quality of life measures are not intuitive

Health-related quality of life is difficult to measure because it is a vague concept with many definitions. Consequently, scores derived from quality of life instruments have no intuitive meaning with few built-in checks or reference values to compare research data against.

For example, by how much does the score of an individual on a quality of life scale have to improve or deteriorate to constitute a meaningful change? This notion of a "minimally important change" is particularly important when evaluating the effect of healthcare. The value for a minimally important change can be calculated by comparing quality of life data against an "anchor".[9] The anchors may be measures of similar concepts, such as global health ratings, or may be related to another situation, such as life events or differences in clinical status.[10] A value for the minimally important change can be derived mathematically and is used to assess the responsiveness of instruments.[11]

Properties of the index

Any index must fulfil several requirements of ease of use and accuracy, etc. (see Chapter 7) but no index is perfect in all respects. Consequently, measures should be selected according to the task in hand. Longitudinal research requires measures that are stable over time and this intra-subject reliability should be established in test-retest studies.[11] A related feature of the index is the ability respond to change. Measures are more responsive to change if most individuals appear to change to the same degree. If the measure records improvements in some patients and deteriorations in others, then it will be difficult to distinguish the effect of the intervention from the variation between individuals.[10,11]

Dealing with missing quality of life data

Missing data is a particular problem in longitudinal research because data missing from one assessment may exclude patients from the entire analysis. Data may be missing as isolated events or (more commonly) because participants leave the study before its completion. The treatment of missing data depends on why it is missing and whether the loss is random or related to the outcome. Methods for preventing and dealing with missing data have been discussed by Curran and colleagues and Fairclough.[9,12]

Multidimensionality of quality of life

The disabilities and handicaps brought about by health problems may impact on many aspects of life. For example, oral health-related quality of life measures assess the impacts related to only a small part of the body, yet consider, among other things, oral pain and the ability to eat, speak, sleep, socialise, perform one's daily duties, and smile.[13] The multidimensional nature of quality of life has profound implications for research (Table 10.1).

Three different approaches are adopted to overcome these implications:

Table 10.1 Implications of a multidimensional concept of quality of life when losing a tooth

Implication	Example
The dimensions affected will differ in different people	The gap will be more visible in some people whereas others will be less able to eat
Health problems can affect many or some dimensions	Some people will be disfigured and less able to eat
The dimensions vary in importance between individuals	Some people will not mind about their appearance
The dimensions vary in importance within individuals	It may be more embarrassing to have a gap when attending a social engagement
Healthcare may replace one impact with another	Losing a painful tooth may make it easier to eat but more embarrassing to smile
Disability in one dimension can be compensated in another	Person may be embarrassed about having a gap but finds solace and balance in his/her ability to eat

- to consider each dimension separately
- to summarise all the dimensions as a single value
- to focus the research on only the relevant dimensions.

Dimensions are treated separately in instruments that profile each individual. By considering the effects on smiling and eating independently, the different effects of losing a tooth described in Table 10.1 can be identified. Against these advantages are the problems brought about by complexity of analysis; not least that analysis of a profile with several dimensions will increase the risk of finding a change by chance alone (type one error).

Data from a multi-item scale can be summarised as a single value (summary measure) in many ways. Typical methods include calculating the number of impacts or a total score that incorporates the frequency or severity of the impacts. Data aggregated in this way are more reliable but will mask any variations between the dimensions (i.e. be less internally consistent and homogeneous).[4] Baseline values and confounders should be considered carefully when analysing summary statistics and the way in which data are summarised will influence the approach used for handling missing data.[9]

Because summary scores ignore the differences between the dimensions and their relative importance to individual participants, more weight can be given to particular dimensions. Weighting factors derived during the development of the instrument are sensitive to the context in which they are used and may require revision if used; for example, in another country.[14] In some cases, the use of item weights does not increase the validity of an instrument.[15,16] Individualised measures allow participants to select or assign their own weights (see Chapter 3).[17] However, neither weighting nor individualisation solve all the problems of summarising data described in Table 10.1.

Perhaps the crudest summary measures are global ratings. Global ratings ask participants to describe their health in a single phrase. For example, the global oral health rating asks "How would you rate your oral health?" with responses on a five-point Likert scale from "excellent" to "poor".[18] A related approach is to use global transition judgements in which participants describe their change in health in a similarly simple way. Not surprisingly, global data ignore the distinctions between the different dimensions of quality of life and are imprecise. However, global judgements provide valid assessments of subjective health status and are often used as gold standards for the construction and validation of new multi-item instruments.[10,19,20]

Using multidimensional and global ratings together has advantages.[21,22] The global ratings can be used to validate the analyses of the individual dimensions and to identify which dimensions contribute most to the change in quality of life.

Other summary measures may be used to capture change. Slade categorised changes in individuals as increments (if impacts at follow up were not reported at baseline), decrements (impacts at baseline not reported at follow up) and net change (impacts at follow up minus the number at baseline, i.e. the increment minus the decrement).[23]

Individuals likely to have changes in quality of life reported increments, decrements, and net change that were not detected in the more typical analyses of group mean scores. In a similar finding, Guyatt and colleagues have extended their concept of a minimally important change to categorise patients who do or do not benefit from treatment.[24] By comparing the proportions of patients who benefited from treatment they were able to discriminate between treatments even though mean differences in quality of life between the treatment groups remained relatively small.

Other approaches to measuring change in quality of life

Two other approaches can be used in longitudinal analysis of quality of life data – repeated measures designs and growth curve models.

Repeated measures designs

Repeated measures designs extend the concept of before and after designs by assessing patients at several stages during the disease or treatment progression.[9] Whilst it is common to analyse the data using independent analyses at each time point, this method does not take into account the fact that scores from the same subjects are dependent on one another. For the same reason, graphs of the average score for each time point do not represent the average profile of the subjects. A better solution is to create a graph for each patient, but this is obviously impractical for more than a handful of participants.[25]

The basic approach to the analysis of repeated measures is to simplify the serial measurements for each subject as a single outcome.[26] This method lends greater power to the analysis and reduces the number of comparisons. Simple outcomes can be calculated, such as the total score or the minimum time to reach the maximum, etc. More complex procedures can be used for each individual subject. For example, a linear regression model could calculate the weekly change in quality of life for each subject. Common statistical procedures that assume independence among the observations can then be applied to the derived values.

Growth curve models

The objective of longitudinal studies is to explore change, generally trends, across time under the same experimental conditions. In growth curve or time course models the main concern is with the shape of response over time. The repeated measurements are in relation to a specified reference point and can accommodate measurements collected at irregular visits.[27] Such models are useful where treatment duration has not been determined in advance, where the quality of life may be affected by changes or events experienced by patients and where there are missing data.[28,29]

Response shift

The concept of response shift theorises that an individual's internal standards or values of assessment may be recalibrated or reconceptualised (see Chapter 2).[2,3] This theory explains the "disability paradox" in which people with severe health problems often report a quality of life that is as good as or better than healthy individuals.

Hard outcome measurements, such as blood pressure or biochemical assays, allow straightforward comparisons over time on a consistently calibrated instrument. Crucially, however, subjective assessments of quality of life may be influenced by the individual's perceptions of health or experience of disease and are notoriously difficult to measure and evaluate.

Three types of change can be characterised: alpha, beta and gamma.[30] Alpha change is that captured by a constantly calibrated instrument in a constant conceptual domain. Beta change occurs in a constant conceptual domain where the intervals of measurement (i.e. the instrument) have been recalibrated. Gamma change involves a reconceptualisation of the domain. These three types of change might be experienced by a woman during labour. Alpha change would be reflected in a series of electrograms of uterine contractions. Self-reported perceptions of pain from these contractions may be susceptible to beta change if the woman's perception of pain is recalibrated. She might say "I didn't know what pain was until I had children". Gamma change would occur if she relegated her pain to a secondary concern as she began to worry about her baby's health.

Response shift complicates analysis by making it difficult to distinguish between changes brought about by treatment or the progression of disease on the one hand and other types of beta and gamma change on the other. For example, older people describe adapting to new situations in order to stay healthy.[31] Similarly, people with chronic illness "normalise" their symptoms in order to reduce their impact, and those with disabilities in one dimension balance the loss or chaos in their lives by compensating in other dimensions (Table 10.1)[22,23,32,33] In a randomised controlled trial any of these changes could mask any potential benefits of treatment.

But an understanding of the dynamic and contextual qualities of response shift also provides important new insights into longitudinal analysis. For example, it allows a distinction to be made between therapies that aim to relieve the intensity of symptoms and those that help patients to cope with symptoms. In such a case, gamma change may reflect a successful outcome of care.

Analytical approaches in the evaluation of response shift

We have seen how the dynamic nature of quality of life presents analytical challenges. A number of possible solutions to these problems have been proposed.[2,34] Some methods require each individual to define, measure or assess the importance of the relevant dimensions of quality of life. Design-based methods use an anchor point or "ideal" scale for reference. Whilst many of these approaches may elucidate aspects of response shift, none will provide a solution to all of the problems it poses. Most of the methods remain unevaluated in quality of life research and many of them place additional burdens on researchers and participants. Moreover, it is difficult to incorporate qualitative data into the quantitative analysis discussed in this chapter.

Evaluating recalibration (beta change)

One method of recalibrating an item or domain is to use a then-test. The baseline value of the conventional before–after comparison is replaced by a retrospective assessment of the baseline, made immediately after the assessment of the after-measurements.

Let us suppose that the woman in the example above rates the intensity of pain on a scale from 1 to 10. Her ratings in early labour were 6 and between contractions in late labour they were also 6. A conventional comparison would infer that the pain intensity was similar. A then-test would ask the woman to recall and rate her pain in early labour ("then"). If the patient recalls the pain in the then-test as 4, we can infer a recalibration of the pain intensity and that her pain intensity has increased by 2 units. The difference between the pre-test and the then-test is the response shift due to scale recalibration.

Evaluating reconceptualisation (gamma change)

Gamma change is a radical redefinition of the structure of the underlying construct that may be detected using factor analysis.[30] Factor analytical techniques can be used to compare the relative influence of a group of variables over time. Any major incongruence between the factorial structures representing each set of questionnaire data, gathered at several points in time, could be interpreted as a change in the dimensions of reality, that is, as gamma change. Golembiewski and colleagues recommended transformation analysis to compare factorial structures. Obviously, nearly fifty years later, more sophisticated methods are available – for example, STATIST, Meta-Biplot and Three Way Principal Components Analysis.[30]

References

1. Locker D. Issues in measuring change in self-perceived oral health status. *Community Dent Oral Epidemiol* 1998;**26**:41–7.
2. Allison PJ, Locker D, Feine JS. Quality of life: a dynamic construct. *Soc Sci Med* 1997;**45**:221–30.
3. Schwartz CE, Sprangers MAG. *Adaptation to changing health. Response shift in Quality-of-Life Research.* Washington: American Psychological Association, 2000.
4. Streiner DL, Norman GR. *Health Measurement Scales,* 2nd ed. Oxford: Oxford University Press, 1995.
5. Cronbach LLF. How should we measure "change" – or should we? *Psychol Bull* 1970;**74**:68–80.
6. Van der Kamp L, Bijleveld CCJH. Methodological issues in longitudinal research. In: Bijleveld CCJH, Van der Kamp LJT, eds. *Longitudinal data analysis.* London: Sage Publications Ltd, 1998, pp. 1–44.
7. Worthington HV. Statistical aspects of measuring change in oral health status of older adults. *Community Dent Oral Epidemiol* 1998;**26**:48–51.
8. Assmann S, Pocock S, Enos L, Kasten L. Subgroup analysis and other (mis)uses of baseline data in clinical trials. *Lancet* 2000;**355**:1064–9.
9. Fairclough D. Methods of analysis for longitudinal studies of health related quality of life. In: Staquet M, Hays R, Fayers P, eds. *Quality of life assessment in clinical trials.* Oxford: Oxford University Press, 1998, pp. 249–80.
10. Guyatt GH. Making sense of quality of life data. *Med Care* 2000; **38**(suppl):II175–9.
11. Guyatt G, Walter S, Norman G. Measuring change over time: assessing the usefulness of evaluative instruments. *J Chronic Disability* 1987;**40**:171–8.
12. Curran D, Fayers P, Molenberghs G, Machin D. Analysis of incomplete quality of life data in clinical trials. In: Staquet M, Hays R, Fayers P, eds. *Quality of life assessment in clinical trials.* Oxford: Oxford University Press, 1998, pp. 227–47.
13. Slade GD, ed. *Measuring oral health and quality of life.* Chapel Hill, NC: University of North Carolina, 1997.
14. Hobart J, Freeman J, Lamping D, Fitzpatrick R, Thompson A. The SF-36 in multiple sclerosis: why basic assumptions must be tested. *J Neurol Neurosurg Psychiatry* 2001;**71**:363–70.
15. Allen FP, Locker D. Do item weights matter? an assessment using the oral health impact profile. *Community Dent Health* 1997;**14**:133–8.
16. Robinson PG, Gibson B, Khan FA, Birnbaum W. Validity of two oral health related quality of life measures in a UK setting. *Community Dent Oral Epidemiol* (in press).

17. Joyce CRB, O'Boyle CA, McGee H. *Individual quality of life. Approaches to conceptualisation and assessment.* Amsterdam: Harwood Academic Publishers, 1999.

18. Atchison KA, Gift HC. Perceived oral health in a diverse sample. *Adv Dent Res* 1997;**11**:272–80.

19. Rowan K. Global questions and scores. In: Jenkinson C, ed. *Measuring health and medical outcomes.* London: UCL Press, 1994.

20. Bowling A. *Measuring health. A review of quality of life measurement scales,* 2nd ed. Buckingham: Open University Press, 1997.

21. Osoba D. Guidelines for measuring health-related quality of life in clinical trials. In: Staquet MJ, Hays RD, Fayers PM, eds. *Quality of life assessment in clinical trials.* Oxford: Oxford University Press, 1998, pp. 19–35.

22. Bernheim J. How to get serious answers to the serious question: "How have you been?": subjective quality of life (QOL) as an individual experiential emergent construct. *Bioethics* 1999;**13**: 272–87.

23. Slade GD. Assessing change in quality of life using the Oral Health Impact Profile. *Community Dent Oral Epidemiol* 1998;**26**:52–61.

24. Guyatt G, Juniper E, Walter S, Griffith L, Goldstein R. Interpreting treatment effects in randomised controlled trials. *BMJ* 1998;**316**:690–93.

25. Everitt BS. *Making sense of statistics in psychology.* Oxford: Oxford University Press, 1996.

26. Mathews JNS, Altman DG, Campbell MJ, Royston P. Analysis of serial measurements in medical research. *BMJ* 1990;**300**:230–35.

27. Zee BC. Growth curve model analysis for quality of life data. *Stat Med* 1998;**17**:757–66.

28. Diggle PJ, Lian KY, Zeger SL. *Analysis of longitudinal studies.* Oxford: Oxford University Press, 1994.

29. Schwartz CE. Teaching coping skills enhances quality of life more than peer support: results of a randomized trial with multiple sclerosis patients. *Health Psychol* 1999;**18**:211–20.

30. Golembiewski RT, Billingsley K, Yeager S. Measuring change and persistence in human affairs: types of change generated by OD designs. *J Appl Behav Sci* 1976;**12**:133–57.

31. MacEntee MI, Hole R, Stolar E. The significance of the mouth in old age. *Soc Sci Med* 1997;**45**:1449–58.

32. Strauss AL, Corbin J, Fagerhaugh S *et al. Chronic illness and the quality of life.* St Louis, MS: CV Mosby, 1984.

33. Albrecht G, Devlieger P. The disability paradox: high quality of life against all the odds. *Soc Sci Med* 1999;**48**:977–88.

34. Schwartz C, Sprangers M. Methodological approaches for assessing response shift in longitudinal health-related quality of life research. *Soc Sci Med* 1999;**48**:1531–48.

11: Is there such a thing as a life not worth living?

BOBBIE FARSIDES AND ROBERT J DUNLOP

Summary points

- There are no quality of life measures that can reliably identify patients who feel that life is not worth living.
- Basing management decisions on such measures requires extreme caution:
  - (a) because of the fluctuating nature of terminally ill or severely disabled patients' valuations of life and desire for death
  - (b) because even patients who are dying may find some quality in life, despite poor objective indicators of quality of life.
- Use of proxies in determining whether a life is worth living is also problematic because of the possible disparity between an observer's assessment of quality of life and the patient's own valuation.
- Nevertheless, patients and proxies (parents) identify health states that they consider to be worse than death.

Introduction

Quality of life measurement has an important place in healthcare. But what about the situation when life has no quality? Or worse? From an ethical perspective, there are two areas in which these issues have been extensively explored: termination of pregnancy, and end of life decision-making for competent and non-competent adults. One particular way in which quality of life is sometimes introduced to decision-making is via the concept of "a life not worth living". The seemingly logical conclusion is that lives not worth living may not be worth creating, saving or preserving. This chapter debates the particular problems (both practical measurement difficulties and ethical issues) associated with quality of life measurement in situations where lives are judged as having no quality.

The beginning and the end

In the case of termination of pregnancy for fetal abnormality, we can never know for sure that the life in question will not be worth living. However, we allow that lives predicted to be of low (or maybe even only slightly diminished) quality, can be terminated. We make these decisions not only or maybe even not primarily because of the judgements of quality but rather because of the morally tenuous status of a biological as opposed to a potentially lived life, and the attendant idea that a fetus' interests can be trumped by those of others. We may also rely on ideas of replaceability (the possibility of creating another biological life) unavailable to us once we judge a lived life to have commenced.

In terms of non-competent adults we have a similar though not as limiting problem with accessing the patient's judgement, but when we feel we can do so we are allowed to rely upon it to decide about non-treatment, etc. However, the fact that someone has lived a life means that we are not entitled to end their life in the interests of others. Their moral status remains undiminished by the deterioration in quality of their lived life, and even a confident assumption that they would not want to carry on living is not taken to justify the direct and intentional termination of their life. In a sense, we commit them to living their biological life in respect for the lived life they may never regain, but we acknowledge that the quality of that lived life may make it unworthy of prolonging or saving.

In terms of the competent adult, we can ascertain whether or not they believe their life to be worth living, but the patient cannot use that claim as the basis for a demand that we should end their lives. Once again the interests of the person are trumped, this time by societal concerns about deliberate killing or individual moral reluctance to end a life. We would not be permitted to end this person's life in the interests of others, but we are permitted to deny them the means to the death they might prefer given their evaluation of its quality.

Who can say that a life is not worth living?

The moral concept of "a life not worth living" raises important quality of life measurement issues. In competent adults who are terminally ill, there are formidable problems in using any quality of life instruments. Many people who arguably are most likely to feel that their own life is not worth living are too ill to complete any quality of life assessments.

Furthermore, few quality of life instruments specifically address this issue. Depression scales often assess suicidal ideation. For example, the Beck Depression Inventory[1] includes specific items: "I feel I would be better off dead", "I feel my family would be better off if I were dead", and "I would kill myself if I could". This emphasises the key role that depression plays in triggering a sense of worthlessness. The implication is that appropriate treatment will reverse this feeling, though some would argue that the beneficial effect of anti-depressant treatments on quality of life has yet to be quantified.[2]

While depression, which is a common feature of terminal illness, may cause a person to feel that life is not worthwhile, it cannot be assumed that patients' requests for death are a proxy for a life not worth living. Chochinov and colleagues[3] found that fleeting or occasional thoughts of a desire for death were common among the terminally ill, but few patients expressed a genuine desire for death. Chochinov and colleauges[4] subsequently found that "will to live" fluctuates substantially in dying patients, particularly in relation to depression, anxiety, shortness of breath, and sense of wellbeing. If "will to live" is inversely related to a sense that "life is not worth living", it could be expected that this sense would also fluctuate over time. While such a relationship is speculative, there is enough doubt to conclude that any study of "life not worth living" must take this into account.

There is evidence suggesting that some patients who think that life is not worth living are not depressed, and it is important to acknowledge such a possibility. Ganzini and colleagues[5] found that patients with motor neurone disease who were willing to consider assisted suicide had higher scores for hopelessness and lower scores for quality of life. Significantly, hopelessness and depression were not synonymous in these patients. However, only one patient expressed a wish for assisted suicide within the next month; it is as if the remaining patients were saying "I can foresee a time when life may not be worth living". Clinical experience would suggest that even the one patient's comment should be interpreted with caution. Sometimes, patients use a request for euthanasia as a cry for help: "life is not worth living now ... but if I could manage (symptom x, problem y or fear of z), then life would still be worth living". However, a patient's evaluation might remain unchanged, even in the face of better care that resulted in the alleviation of painful or traumatic symptoms.

Some patients do persist in requests for euthanasia and follow through these requests. Prospective quality of life studies have not been carried out with these patients. Chin and colleagues[6] found retrospective evidence from physicians to suggest that patients who actually commit assisted suicide were more likely to be concerned about loss of autonomy and loss of control of bodily functions. The assumption[7] that depression was not a contributory factor for these patients cannot be sustained from this study, but the message is none the less important. In a recent study conducted in the Netherlands, physicians reported "avoiding loss of dignity" and "unbearable or hopeless suffering" as the two most common reasons for patients requesting euthanasia.[8]

The limitations of current measures

Studies have not indicated any objective way of clearly identifying patients who would feel that life is not worth living. Patients may even find quality in life when imminently dying, when their quality of life assessed by current measures is abysmal.[9] This calls into question any notion that observers can reliably judge if and when incompetent adults might have considered life to be not worthwhile. Proxy measures of quality of life, by relatives or healthcare professionals, for example, frequently underestimate patients' quality of life.[10] Emanuel and Emanuel[11] also found that family members and proxies often do not accurately know what a patient's values or preferences might be, casting doubt on their ability to make decisions for incompetent patients. The use of proxies to measure quality of life was discussed in detail in Chapter 6.[12]

In relation to termination of pregnancy, the impact of an abnormal lived life has been explored by Boyle and colleagues.[13] They did not assess the effects of fetal abnormalities. However, they evaluated the medium-term impact of very low birth weight in a cohort of survivors from a regional neonatal intensive care programme. The study used the Health Utilities Index (HUI), a variant of the quality-adjusted life years (QALY) methodology. QALYs attempt to aggregate both quality and duration of life data into a single outcome measure, which can then be used to describe the benefit of a particular healthcare programme or technology.[14] The benefit measure is then divided by the cost of the programme, resulting in a ratio that can be used to allocate resources.[15]

Boyle and colleagues[13] created a classification of health states using quality of life domains: physical function, role function, social and emotional function, and health problems. Each domain was sub-divided into different levels, giving rise to 960 possible combinations. Each combination represented a distinct possible health state. A random sample of parents then created a ranking of these health states by comparing the desirability/undesirability of each health state with other health states and with the reference states "healthy" and "dead". By assigning the values 1 to "healthy" and 0 to "dead", each health state could theoretically be assigned a value between 0 and 1. In practice, the investigators found that parents ranked some chronic dysfunctional states in children as worse than death.

Following on from the concerns about healthy proxies judging the quality of life of others, some patients have been involved in ranking health states. For example, Rosser and Kind[16] used psychiatric and medical patients, as well as healthy volunteers and healthcare professionals. These patients also ranked some health states as worse than death, notably the states of being confined to bed in severe distress and unconscious in no distress. However, the use of "death" as an anchor point can make some subjects reluctant to answer and thereby produce arbitrary results.[15] The EuroQol questionnaire avoids this by using "worst imaginable health state" as the negative anchor point.[17] It is not clear how this relates to "life not worth living".

QALYs are the best known but not the only approach to the economic analysis of quality of life and survival data.[14] These methodologies can result in a different but profound interpretation of "life not worth living", namely that particular lives may have a detrimental economic worth. Moral as well as technical concerns inevitably surround this field of work,[14,15,18] not least being the concern that the methods of assessing quality of life values from individuals does not reflect the use to which they will be put.[15] However, it is clear that these methodologies will play an increasing role in health technology assessment and resource allocation.

Discussion and future directions

Ultimately, all three examples show little effective role for the concept of a life not worth living. In the case of termination of pregnancy, it is because it is unclear how we would establish the claim, and what is more it is unnecessary, given the attitudes we have adopted to the limited moral status of the healthy fetus. In the second and third cases, the moral status of the person who has lived and in some cases is still living their (lived) life rules out the possibility of trumping their interest in being alive to the extent that we could not kill them in the interest of others. However, our wish to endorse the importance of that moral prohibition means that we will trump their interests when they claim that they want to die. Thus the idea that the life is not worth living has little power other than in supporting a non-treatment decision that will prevent a life being prolonged or saved. Whilst the moral, social, and political reasons for wanting to maintain a prohibition upon ending lived lives are powerful, it is important to acknowledge the way in which this denies individuals the right to make the full range of choices which logically follow from a decision that life is not worth living.

Acknowledgements

We thank our colleagues in the Interdisciplinary Research Group in Palliative and Person Centred Care at King's College, London, in particular Irene Higginson, Alison Carr, Peter Robinson, Barry Gibson, Stanley Gelbier, Julia Addington-Hall, Lalit Kalra, and Alan Turner-Smith, who have participated in discussions and commented on an earlier draft of this work.

References

1. Beck AT, Ward CH, Mendelson M *et al*. An inventory for measuring depression. *Arc Gen Psychiatry* 1961;**4**:561–71.
2. Orley J, Saxena S, Herrman H. Quality of life and mental illness: reflections from the perspective of the WHOQOL. *Br J Psychiatry* 1998;**172**:291–3.
3. Chochinov HM, Wilson KG, Enns M *et al*. Desire for death in the terminally ill. *Am J Psychiatry* 1995;**152**:1185–91.
4. Chochinov HM, Tataryn D, Clinch JJ *et al*. Will to live in the terminally ill. *Lancet* 1999;**354**:816–19.
5. Ganzini L, Johnston WS, McFarland BH *et al*. Attitudes of patients with amyotrophic lateral sclerosis and their care givers toward assisted suicide. *N Engl J Med* 1998;**339**:967–73.
6. Chin AE, Hedberg K, Higginson GK *et al*. Legalized physician-assisted suicide in Oregon – the first year's experience. *N Engl J Med* 1999;**340**:577–83.
7. Enck RE. Recent issues in physician-assisted suicide. *Am J Hosp Palliative Care* 1999;**16**:500–501.
8. Haverkate I, Onwuteaka-Philipsen BD, van der Heide A *et al*. Refused and granted requests for euthanasia and assisted suicide in the Netherlands: interview study with structured questionnaire. *BMJ* 2000;**321**:865–6.
9. Mount BM, Scott JS. Whither hospice evaluation? *J Chronic Dis* 1983;**36**:731–6.
10. Sprangers MAG, Aaronson NK. The role of health care providers and significant others in evaluating the quality of life of patients with chronic disease: a review. *J Clin Epidemiol* 1992;**45**:743–60.
11. Emanuel EJ, Emanuel LL. Proxy decision-making for incompetent patients: an ethical and empirical analysis. *JAMA* 1992;**267**: 2067–71.
12. Addington-Hall J, Kalra L. Who should measure QoL? *BMJ* 2001;**322**:1417–20.

13. Boyle MH, Torrance GW, Sinclair JC *et al*. Economic evaluation of neonatal intensive care of very-low-birth-weight infants. *N Engl J Med* 1983;**308**:1330–37.

14. Billingham LJ, Abrams KR, Jones DR. Methods of analysis of quality-of-life and survival data in health technology assessment. *Health Technol Assess* 1999;**3**:55–63.

15. Spiegelhalter DJ, Gore SM, Fitzpatrick R *et al*. Quality of life measures in health care. III: resource allocation. *BMJ* 1992;**305**:1205–9.

16. Rosser R, Kind P. A scale of valuations of states of illness: is there a social consensus? *Int J Epidemiol* 1978;**7**:347–58.

17. van Agt HME, Essink-Bot ML, Krabbe PFM *et al*. Test-retest reliability of health state valuations collected with the EuroQol questionnaire. *Soc Sci Med* 1994;**39**:1537–44.

18. Kaplan RM. Profile versus utility based measures of outcome for clinical trials. In: Staquet MJ, Hays RD, Fayers PM, eds. *Quality of life assessment in clinical trials: methods and practice*. Oxford, Oxford University Press, 1998, pp. 69–92.

Glossary

Accuracy: the degree to which measurements are correct.

Alpha change: occurs when the conceptual domain (for example, what constitutes quality of life for the individual) remains constant over time, and the way in which it is rated or calibrated also remains constant over time. This "ideal" state is the underlying assumption for all current statistical assessments of change in quality of life over time, or following a treatment intervention.

Back translation: when a measure is adapted for use in another language, it is first translated into the second language, and then this second version is translated back into the original language to ensure that it is still equivalent.

Beta change: occurs when the conceptual domain remains constant over time, but the individual's internal assessment of how good or bad it is is recalibrated. In other words, a QoL score of six at one time point, may equate to a score of nine at a second time point.

Ceiling effects: occur when the measure is unable to detect an improvement in QoL in people who generally have a good quality of life. It is usually related to the design of the measure (the items and the scaling systems used).

Conceptual equivalence: when the underlying concept as represented by the measure is the same in the different populations in which the measure is being used. For example, are the determinants of quality of life the same in Africa as in USA.

Constructs: underlying psychological perceptions or definitions.

Construct validity: when the attribute or construct being measured is not directly observable, and there are no gold standard measures against which the new measure can be tested (criterion validity), construct validity is assessed. This involves testing a series of hypotheses in order to see whether the new scale relates to other variables in the expected way.

Content validity: the extent to which the domains and level of questions are appropriate for the setting and participants being studied. For example, have the full range of questions that capture QoL relating to cancer been included and is the scaling or scoring system constructed so that the full range of severities can be measured.

Criterion validity: the extent to which a questionnaire measures what it claims to measure as assessed by comparison with a gold standard measure of the same attribute.

Cronbach's alpha: a statistic that is an indication of the internal consistency of a measure. It assesses the degree to which all the items in a questionnaire measure the same underlying construct.

Disability: difficulty or the inability to perform activities as a result of a medical condition that would be considered normal for someone of the same age.

Disability paradox: where patients who clearly have significant health and functional problems or intrusive symptoms nevertheless have high QoL scores.

Discriminative measures: measures designed to discriminate between groups of patients.

Disease-specific health-related QoL scales: measures designed to capture the particular QoL issues relating to specific anatomic divisions, body systems or diseases.

Domains: different aspects of QoL that might be included in a questionnaire. For example, pain, function, social interaction, emotional wellbeing, work and so on are domains.

Evaluative measures: assess change over time, for example, in a randomised controlled trial.

Factor analysis: a mathematical technique used to develop scales that measure a single characteristic or attribute. Factor analysis can be used to determine which items and subscales belong to which underlying "factor" of a construct such as QoL. It also determines the strength of the statistical relationship between factors and leads to the elimination of items that bear a weak relationship to the factor with which they should relate and items that contribute little to the overall questionnaire score.

Floor effects: occur when the measure is unable to detect deterioration in people who already have a poor QoL.

Gamma change: occurs when the conceptual domain alters (for example, what constitutes QoL for the individual changes) *and* the individual's internal assessment of how good or bad it is, is recalibrated.

Generalisability: describes the degree to which the items in a questionnaire or its psychometric properties are relevant to populations other than those in which the questionnaire was devised.

Generic health-related QoL scales: are broad measures of QoL that contain items of relevance to most people, irrespective of specific anatomical divisions, body systems or diseases.

Global ratings: are summary measures of an attribute such as QoL and usually only consist of one question. For example, "Considering all the ways in which your condition affects you, how would you rate your quality of life today?".

Global transition judgements: are summary assessments of how much the attribute has changed.

Handicap: is the degree to which a person is disadvantaged in terms of their social interactions, role fulfilment and participation as a result of their medical condition.

Indices: are questionnaires that provide a single summary score.

Individualised measures: individualised measures of QoL try to assess the individual patient's construct of QoL, rather than asking them to rate their QoL against a set of predetermined items. For example, some QoL measures ask patients to specify those aspects of life that are important to them (as an open question) and then rate the impact of their condition on those areas.

Internal consistency: is the degree to which the items in a questionnaire all measure the same attribute. It is a form of reliability and is important for questionnaires that measure one dimensional attributes such as depression.

Item: usually refers to one question on a questionnaire.

Item impact method: selects items for inclusion in a questionnaire not on the basis of their relationship to one another (as in the case of factor analysis), but on the basis of their importance to patients.

Item weights: many scales use a weighting method to enhance the sensitivity of the questionnaire. This involves the allocation of greater weights to items that are more important to the overall end score. For example, if independence were found to be more important to patients than body image, the questionnaire item(s) relating to independence would be given a greater weighting than the body image items. This means that the item will have more of an influence upon the final QoL score. There are several methods for generating item weights.

Intrasubject reliability: often termed inter-rater reliability, this is the degree of consistency with which questionnaires behave when applied to different people. If the same patient is being assessed by two different observers, under the same conditions, the results from the administered questionnaire should be the same.

Minimally important change: the smallest detectable change in a questionnaire score (that is, greater than the measurement error) that is considered important either by the clinician, the researcher or the patient.

Normalise: the process of reinterpreting symptoms so that they are not viewed as indicative of disease or illness.

Participation: the ability to engage in society or to fulfil roles that are normal for age and background.

Predictive measures: classify individuals into categories predefined by existing criteria. For example, when screening for disease.

Profile: a questionnaire that provides several subscores that cannot be amalgamated into a single numerical score (usually because they represent distinct attributes or entities). An example is the SF-36 that provides separate scores for function, vitality, emotional role, social role and so on.

Proxy: someone who completes a questionnaire on behalf of the intended subject because of their inability to complete it (for example, because of cognitive impairment or because they are too young).

Proxy measures: are substitute measures of an attribute that are used when it is not possible to measure the attribute directly.

Psychometric properties: are the measurement properties of a questionnaire and generally refer to its validity, reliability, responsiveness and appropriateness.

Recall bias: occurs when memory distorts the assessment or perception of an attribute.

Reference period: the time period over which questionnaires measure an attribute. For example, some questionnaires ask about the last three months, some ask about the last week and others ask for a momentary assessment.

Reliability: is the consistency with which a questionnaire measures what it is designed to measure. For example, does it produce the same results when repeated in the same population.

Responsiveness: (also called sensitivity) the ability of the questionnaire to detect meaningful change.

Response shift: refers to a change in the meaning of self evaluation of a particular outcome and can occur as the result of two factors:

a) A change in the patient's internal standards of measurement. In other words, a recalibration of their scale for that outcome. For example, a VAS pain score of 63mm before treatment may equate to a pain score of 88mm after treatment because the patient's expectations of pain relief have altered.

b) A redefinition of the outcome by the patient. For example, the symptom described as pain becomes something different or those factors constituting QoL change.

Semantic equivalence: the degree to which questionnaires that have been translated into secondary languages, mean/ask the same thing as the original questionnaire. Back translation is used to ensure semantic equivalence.

Standardised measures: questionnaires that ask every respondent the same set of questions and require them to choose from the same set of predefined responses or scales.

Test retest reliability: the degree to which a questionnaire gives the same results when administered to the same individual, under the same conditions on more than one occasion. The time period over which the repeated administrations are made is selected to ensure that the individual has not changed with respect to the attribute being measured, whilst being sufficiently distant for them not to be able to simply memorise their previous responses to the questionnaire.

Then-tests: used to assess whether response shift has occurred. This involves asking patients to make baseline and post treatment assessments and then to make post-treatment, retrospective assessments of baseline health status using the same outcome measure. These retrospective then-tests should be performed at the same time as the conventional post-treatment assessments. The assumption is that the then-tests will be based on the same internal calibration and conceptualisation of the outcome as the conventional post-treatment assessment. Any difference between the conventional baseline measure and the then-test is assumed to be due to response shift. Whilst the simplicity of this method is attractive, it is limited by the potential problem of recall bias.

Type one error: the probability of detecting a significant difference when the treatments are really equally effective.

Validity: is the degree to which the questionnaire measures what it is designed to measure. There are several different types of validity: face, content, criterion, construct, discriminant and convergent.

Index